FROM DISA
TO ENABLED

Our story of transformation and
restoration of body, mind and soul

Mike Denton

Charmaine O'Reilly

Foreword by

Jules Kelly

Claire Morton

Jessica Cunningham

Content

FOREWORD

"Purpose"

Definition:

The reason for which something is done or created or for which something exists.

"the purpose of the meeting is to appoint a trustee"

a person's sense of resolve or determination.

"there was a new **sense of purpose** in her step as she set off"

Somewhere between 2006 and 2017 I lost who I thought I once was. Fibromyalgia stripped me of my freedom, my joy, my ability to be purposeful in any way.

The purpose of this book is to share with those that may be feeling the same way, that there is hope beyond the pain that you or a loved one may be experiencing right now.

Having made a life changing decision in 2017 following a full mental and physical breakdown, that my life could not continue in this way, I decided to take back control of my body and my overall wellbeing.

I realised that I had become a passenger in my own life and that I was no longer driving the bus. I had readily handed the keys over to the medics and the medication that they prescribed. Our society is blessed in many ways that we have medicines available and scientific advances to support the fight for disease.

Somewhere during evolution and the growth of society through the many revolutions of change, we have lost the knowledge of how best to look after our own body. Slowly but surely we have looked for short cuts on how to live life better, faster, easier....all of which generally come with chemicals that are known to disrupt our body systems and the way in which our body innately knows to heal itself.

Our healthcare system is really a sick care system. We visit the doctors' surgery when we are sick. We present with symptoms and their role is, in part to prescribe medication that is licenced to treat the symptom. It's the way my generation have grown up. You have a headache, and you take a tablet. Medication is often the first line of defence. It was for me too until I was 47 years old.

My decision took me on a journey of learning. I learned about the basic functionality of my body. How it works in its simplest form. What affected the way it worked. It led me to swapping out all my opiate pain medication for natural alternatives and it made me really aware of what I was putting in and on to my body.

I learned about my cellular health. I learned about nutrition, and I learned about metaphysics and the impact that life events, lifestyle and trauma have on the body. I became a qualified aromatherapist along with several other qualifications.

(In Human Design I am a 5/1 Manifesting Generator. The 1 represents my need to learn and understand things fully, hence the need to become qualified in the work that I do if it lights me up.)

Removing the medication from my body had a positive impact for me and made no difference to the pain that I was feeling. My mind became clearer, and I was able to embark on counselling and psychotherapy to work through the mental challenges that I had. I found that as I worked through the trauma and all of the emotional and mental challenges, the physical pain started to leave my body.

By the time I was 48 I didn't recognise the woman that I was a year before.

I felt frustrated that the system only supported a medicated response to this condition that almost 3 million people in the UK are living with. Worldwide the number is so much higher (8-10% of the US population)

The Life Audit and Radical Self Care Programme was borne, and this was followed up with The Fading Woman® book. Both document my journey from being disabled to being well again. I created a self-help programme and the book to help others follow the same steps that I did if they chose to.

This process has been refined and strengthened by the introduction of Belief Coding®, meditation programmes and belief education as created by Jessica Cunningham and Claire Morton. Both are Global leading professionals in the holistic world and bringing them in to the newly named Life Freedom Method® is testament to the power and belief that this method will help to change millions of lives.

Fast forward to 2022 and I was invited to share my story on

International Fibromyalgia Day for Cheshire Police. At the event I met a Consultant of Pain Medicine and one of the lead authors of new guidelines for the diagnosis of fibromyalgia syndrome which was launched by the Royal College of Physicians in Liverpool. We took the conversation offline, and he said that he was intrigued by how I could rid myself of the pain. He invited me to bring some patients to his clinical trial by way of an introductory pilot for The Life Freedom Method®.

Mike and Charmaine were the people that I introduced to the trial. They met with the team at The Walton Centre where they were approved for the trial and had lab tests and blood tests taken. They were then passed back to me to start working with them with The Life Freedom Method®

This is their story.

Mike

Hi, I am Mike Denton.

I am a 40-year-old father of three, a husband, and for the past 7 years have been an active serving Police Officer with Cheshire Constabulary.

I am going to share with you my story of life with Fibromyalgia Syndrome, including my life beforehand, being diagnosed, what I have done since then and my plans for the future.

I was born in Leeds and have three siblings. I would say that I had a great childhood. I remember going on family holidays and being out with friends and I have some wonderful memories.

My career journey has been varied and I've had a few jobs over the years starting out with being a cleaner, then working behind a bar, working in an office and working for a bank. These all brought the usual levels of stress but nothing that I would particularly class as high level.

When I was asked to reflect on any trauma that I may have been aware of, apart from a couple of relationship break ups and being knocked down by a car when I was 17 on a crossing, I would consider myself as not really having experienced any trauma.

I now know that trauma doesn't need to be a huge cataclysmic event as I, and probably many others would perceive it, but it can be anything that causes a level of psychological and emotional harm. Everyone is different and something as small as being told to be quiet at school could have a lasting impact.

So, I guess being knocked down was a traumatic experience!

I was on my way home from a volunteer role that I had with Leeds United when a car ran a red light and hit me on my left side throwing me into the air. I remember the passenger getting out and asking if I was ok and me saying "Do I look ok, you just ran me over?".

I asked them to call an ambulance and I called my mum to let her know that I wouldn't be home for tea. The ambulance came and took me to the hospital. The Paramedic asked me if I was a rugby player. He said that if my thighs weren't the size, they were I would have probably broken my pelvis. Luckily, I hadn't broken anything!

In 2003 I moved to North Wales and a few years later got married and life was good. 2008 turned in to a traumatic year for me as my wife and I separated, my son was born at 27 weeks' gestation weighing just 2lbs 5oz and my dad was diagnosed with bowel cancer all within a few short weeks.

I met my beautiful wife Tara and moved to Chester where I began a foundation degree in Policing. Policing was a career that I wanted since I was young. I had applied to different forces over the years but had not been successful, so thought this may be a better way to get to achieve my dream job. I was a Special (volunteer) constable at first and worked in Cheshire Police Head Quarters in the Firearms Licensing department before I became a PC. Over the last ten years I would say that I have witnessed a lot, from drunken fights, neighbour disputes, escapee cows, domestic abuse, people self-harming and experiencing mental health crisis, road traffic collisions, and death.

Several jobs stick in my mind.

I was called to a young lad that cut his wrists in front of me with a steak knife. He had it hidden under a bag. I managed to wrestle it from him and got him to the hospital where his injuries were seen to, and he was given a mental health assessment.

I was called to attend a young girl who was sat on a railway bridge. I managed to talk her down and she was taken back to the hospital that she had just hours before been released from. After a debrief with my superior, whilst driving I spotted the same young girl again walking back towards the train station. I followed her and got out of the car to see her running up to the platform where she climbed back on to the bridge again and jumped.

The cot death of a three-month-old little girl three weeks after my own daughter was born was a difficult job to attend.

To say that these things didn't affect me would be a lie but I have the emotional range of a teaspoon or so I'm told. The reality is these "jobs" are all traumatic incidents that I have witnessed. I'm conditioned to just get on with it.

The reason I am telling you my life story and speaking about trauma is this.

In May of 2019 I had been on a late shift as a Response Officer. I got home in the early hours and went to bed, waking up in the night with excruciating stomach pain.

I was unable to go to work for the following two days as the pain didn't go away. I went to see my GP who referred me to a Gastroenterologist who ran all the tests that you can think of, but they all produced a negative result.

Still unable to work, a couple of weeks later my daughter brought me a bottle of lemonade and asked if I could open it.

I couldn't.

I couldn't move my arms and had no strength in my hands, and I couldn't grip the lid. Let me tell you that it's quite scary when you try to do something you have done forever, and your arms and hands don't work.

I went back to my GP whom by this time I was on first-name terms with. They had me complete a questionnaire on my pain and other symptoms that I was displaying which had spread to various parts of my body. They questioned the position, intensity and frequency and at this point said that they thought I may have Fibromyalgia.

I was referred to a Rheumatologist who requested another myriad of tests and I had to wait to see what if anything was found. My mental health suffered, and it got to the stage where I didn't want to carry on. The pain was constant. I was tired, grumpy, and the pain engulfed my whole body, my fingers, wrists, arms, shoulders, back, legs, feet, literally everywhere and I was generally miserable. I realised that I had my family for support, something to keep going for.

I was referred to Occupational Health who said that I wasn't fit for work. I was sat at home feeling lost and in pain. My supervisor at the time took me out for a catch-up and told me I looked depressed and made another Occupational Health referral with a request to attend the Police Treatment Centre in Harrogate on their two-week Mental Health Wellbeing Course. It was brilliant and something that I cannot speak more highly of. I cannot thank the charity enough for the work that they do for Police Officers.

MIKE II

In July 2021 I finally received the diagnosis of Fibromyalgia after 18 months of hospital appointments, blood tests, x-ray, ultrasounds, CT, and MRI Scans. On the one hand, it was great to finally have a diagnosis, something that I could use to look for answers but on the other hand, Shit!

I have Fibromyalgia, a chronic pain condition, brilliant. I started on medication – Gabapentin which I took for a while but found that I felt no different, so the GP changed this to Pregabalin. I was also prescribed an anti-depressant and painkillers.

I returned to work gradually on reduced hours. Occupational Health was still telling me that I wasn't fit but my pay was about to stop so I didn't really have a choice. I was to be office based so the dream of being a cop out on the streets was gone. Then COVID-19 struck. I started to work from home a couple of hours a day looking through colleagues' workloads to see where I could help then would usually need to sleep in the afternoon as I was so exhausted.

As COVID-19 eased I went back into the office and started a new desk-based role. At this point I shared an office with a Detective Inspector who asked if I had heard of Enable the Disability and Carers network in force. I hadn't but sent an email introducing myself and asking if there was any advice, they could give me on any reasonable adjustments and if there was a Fibromyalgia network.

A couple of days later I received a reply from the Chairperson of the network, Jenny saying that there wasn't a specific network for Fibro, however, I could speak to her as she also had Fibromyalgia. It has been more common for women to be diagnosed with Fibro however Jenny put me in contact with two other male colleagues who had also had a recent diagnosis of Fibromyalgia.

At this point we did not know how many people in the Constabulary suffered from Fibromyalgia, however, I spoke with them and suggested having a network for anyone with Fibro or their friends, family, and carers to join to share advice and have somewhere to ask for support.

I sent emails to the well-being departments of all constabularies across the UK and Ireland asking if any of them had anything similar aimed at specifically supporting employees with Fibromyalgia. I received several replies but apart from one or two the answer was that they didn't.

On the 12th of May 2022 (International Fibromyalgia awareness day) I launched the Fibromyalgia network and I managed to bring some guest speakers together for an online presentation summit where there was an open invite to anyone from any constabulary to attend.

The first speaker was Des Quinn, the Chair of Fibromyalgia Action UK, a charity based in Scotland that offers support and advice to people with Fibro and their friends, family and their employers. Their website FMAUK.co.uk has lots of useful support documents and the staff there are available to assist with any problems that people are facing.

The next speaker David runs a local Facebook Group "Rock Off Fibro" (You can search this on Facebook). David is a carer for his wife who has Fibro and he spoke about how he campaigns to raise awareness of the condition; he has managed to organise artists from around the world to donate songs which were created into a CD raising further awareness.

Dr Andreas Goebel of the Walton Pain Clinic was the next speaker. Dr Goebel is performing research into understanding Fibromyalgia as an auto-immune disease. The research that his team is undertaking may hopefully change the way that Fibromyalgia is viewed and help to develop new ways in which it can be treated.

The final guest speaker was the author of "The Fading Woman", holistic performance, life & business consultant, Jules Kelly. Jules shared how she suffered from Fibromyalgia and designed the Life Freedom Method® enabling her to holistically free herself from the pain that Fibromyalgia brings.

Following the launch of the network I received many emails from officers and staff asking to become members of the support group and a WhatsApp group was set up to allow each of the members to speak with and support each other through their Fibro journeys.

This all gave me an enormous sense of pride and purpose, that I had been able to raise awareness of the condition amongst police forces and be able to offer support to others going through the same things I was. People who don't have the condition don't know what it's like to be in constant pain. Often people with Fibro are thought to be making it up and lazy but that couldn't be farther from the truth. They are fighters, they are Fibro Warriors.

MIKE III

I heard from Jules again who told me that following the web event, she had spoken with Andreas Goebel who had invited her to join his research trial and asked if I would like to be part of the study. Of course, I jumped at the chance. It would involve visiting Andreas' team at the Walton Centre for them to run some tests, these would be blood tests, pressure tests and questions about my health, pain etc. After this, I would be working with Jules for three months using the Life Freedom Method® to hopefully reduce the pain and symptoms of Fibromyalgia and see if the method affected the antibody link that Dr Goebel's team was researching.

There were to be others on the trial, and I was asked if anyone else from the network would like to volunteer that were able to fit the trial criteria. This is where I met the wonderful Charmaine O'Reilly.

We met with Jules in early November 2022 at the Headquarters of Cheshire Constabulary where we chatted through what to expect from the process. Jules ensured that we wanted to get better above everything and would do whatever it took.

We started off by drinking at least 2 litres of water daily and took bioavailable supplements to nourish our bodies. Jules shared the analogy of a fern plant with us. If you give the fern water, good plant food and sunshine it will grow and flourish, if you feed it fizzy soda and fast food, and subject it to the wrong environment, well pretty soon it's going to wither and that is the same with the body.

This resonated with me as I've gone through a stage of eating a lot of fast food, partly I suppose being a response cop you don't really get time to eat a balanced nutritious diet and grab what you can whilst on the go, that is if you get chance to. There's also the fact that being in pain for the last several months, feeling depressed and comfort eating, not wanting to stand and cook something due to the intense pain in my feet and then there's just being lazy and disorganised.

Jules also provided us with a range of essential oils bespoke to what symptoms we were each experiencing. These are all-natural and can be mixed and rubbed into the body and have many properties. Some support the reduction of pain, some the immune system, some mood, some sleep, and so on. As an aromatherapist, Jules created the blends that would best suit each of us.

Once we understood and agreed that we would do anything that it took to get better Jules began to guide us into the Life Freedom Method®.

Well, I'm going to stop just there.

I looked at Jules like she had three heads and had taken illicit substances before meeting with us.

You see there are lots of simple practical steps to it, but we were also to work with the subconscious mind.

We learned about how the subconscious mind stores everything it has ever experienced including trauma. The trauma that you have gone through not only in this life but in the womb and sometimes passed lives too as the soul can carry with it seven generations of trauma.

The process starts with using a kinesiology technique called The Human Compass®. It helps to pinpoint which emotion is held in the part of the body that feels the pain or discomfort. This emotion then helps us to pinpoint any reflection of trauma. The Human Compass® is the technique that allows us to have the subconscious answer to the posed question by identifying a yes and no response with the body.

At this point, I asked Jules if we would also be doing yoga with goats and drinking our own piss but apparently, we wouldn't be doing any of that however one other thing she did recommend we do is journal. Write about our day, how we felt, why we felt like it, and to get things out into the world rather than keeping them trapped inside. We also started on a 14-day meditation course with the lovely Claire Morton who is Jules' business partner. I have tried meditation before using both guided meditation which I did whilst at the PTC in Harrogate and mindfulness meditation using an app. I did these on and off but never carried on with them as my mind wanders off. Claire however got me to pick a mantra to use throughout the sessions to bring my mind back from wandering which was a real help.

Jules also shared our Human Design with us. Jules describes this on her site Spaceandfreedom.com as "a synthesis of a number of modern and ancient systems that are grounded in science that provides us with a soul map of YOU". By entering your date, time, and place of birth your design will tell you your purpose, your strengths, and desires and essentially all about your personality, traits, and characteristics. There are five designs and several centres within the design that carry energy flow where it travels to the throat in order to be communicated. I am a Generator. Generators are creators and have powerful and consistent energy, this allows them to respond to opportunities and challenges and inspires them to accomplish great achievements and bring things to reality, hence starting the Fibro Network. Along with this I have a defined Sacral meaning that I have the ability to gain proficiency in a subject quickly, am creative and have the ability to learn. When I heard this, it resonated with me as I have always found that if something lights me up, I can learn about it quite easily, however, it's the complete opposite if I'm not lit up by what I am doing I can then feel like my energy drains out of me.

The strategy in my Human Design is to respond. This is essentially saying how I interact with life and different scenarios. I tend to have a gut feeling about something whether that be an expansive feeling if something feels right or a contracting feeling if it doesn't, which has always helped in my career as a Police Officer.

I will also use a lot of "Uh Huh" and "Mmmmm" for yes and "Errr" and "Ugh" for no during conversation. I also have a defined root centre meaning that I can kickstart projects and take action, although I also know when it's time to move, something else that I have found over the last 40 years. Along with this, my ego centre is also defined (my wife would probably agree). A defined ego centre means that I know what I want and how to get it. I think I need to master this a bit more but at this point in my life I think that I am on the way to getting there. It's having the motivation to achieve, embrace your self-worth and expression and not just look after the collective but to look after what you want as well.

This was all very interesting but one thing that I found quite thought-provoking was that I have both an undefined ajna and solar plexus centre. The ajna indicates that I am open-minded which again being a Police Officer has come in handy, but it also means that I am designed to contemplate and don't naturally store information meaning that the current school system may not have worked for me. I'm not saying that it didn't work as I did my best and got decent grades, but it was a bit of a struggle at times, and I find that I learn better by someone showing me or telling me how to do something rather than reading about it in a book. The solar plexus centre is all about emotions and feelings and I am able to easily feel other people's emotions. This makes me extremely empathic, and I gain wisdom through exploring this emotional connection. I believe that we are still at a time when society doesn't respond to processing information through emotion, and we tend to use the term "I think" rather than "I feel" due to conditioning. Opening to feelings has really helped me on this journey.

MIKE IV

Jessica Cunningham created Belief Coding®. Jules was one of the first Belief Coding® facilitators in the World and brought the modality and Jessica into The Life Freedom Method® due to its fast targeted results.

Belief Coding® allows the subconscious to revisit past trauma and re-code new beliefs to allow you to move on and change any life-limiting beliefs that may be holding you back.

I am the biggest cynic but was open to the process. During one session with Jules, I was working on the pain in my shoulders. My Human Compass® had identified the emotion that was linked to it as loss.

As we started to belief code, I closed my eyes and I saw a young boy. He was standing next to what appeared to be waves on a shoreline. His name was George, and he was seven years old, and we were in Weatherby near York. He felt lost as his mother who was called Mary had passed away from drowning. His father was a carpenter and was at work, but he was with his Uncle John, oh and the year was 1642.

For George to feel better I asked him what he needed, and he wanted to go to the park, so off we went, he met some friends there and played and felt much better. We coded in new beliefs and like magic the pain that I had suffered for months in my shoulder had eased, I get a twinge every now and again, but the difference is exponential.

I have had a number of emotions that have come through from previous lives and by re-coding the beliefs I have been able to significantly reduce the level of pain that I suffered through Fibromyalgia.

Since then, I have been back to the Walton Centre to see Dr Goebel's team and had the initial tests rerun. You will be able to read the results towards the end of this book.

Looking forward to the future I have attended a Belief Coding® Facilitators course delivered by the inspiring Jessica Cunningham and am at this time training to become accredited in Belief Coding® facilitation. My hope is that I can use this, plus the information that I have learned about taking better care of myself to help others in similar situations throughout the Emergency Services and beyond.

Thank you for taking the time to read about me and my journey and I hope that it may help to show that there are others out there with the same condition but there's also a light at the end of the tunnel.

Mike.

Charmaine

"You have Fibromyalgia".

I was diagnosed in 2017 with this condition called Fibromyalgia. I didn't know anything about it. I assumed it was like the flu due to the symptoms I had, extreme fatigue, pain everywhere, fuzzy head, trouble sleeping and several other irritating symptoms. My first thought was phew, a bout of antibiotics will sort this out. It had been lingering for years so antibiotics were the first thing on my mind.

The doctor laughed when I mentioned antibiotics and gave me some reading material on Fibro. I went home and started reading the stuff on this horrific condition. The things I read made me feel like giving up immediately. Automatically I climbed into bed, put my electric blanket on and told my family they would have to sort out dinner as I felt too unwell to do anything.

The first things that came up when I googled Fibromyalgia were:

A disorder that affects muscle and soft tissue characterised by chronic muscle pain, tenderness, fatigue and sleep disturbances.

A lifelong condition

Common for ages 35-50

More common in females

Treatments can help manage condition, no known cure.

Now, I know I am a bit of a drama queen but when you know

nothing about a condition you have been diagnosed with and you read that you instantly think the worst. I know I did. I burst out crying and thought, HOLY SHIT my life is over!

My name is Charmaine O'Reilly. I am a mother to three beautiful children (adults now but they will always be my babies) and a beautiful little angel in heaven. I am the wife to a crazy dude Trev who has been my support throughout this nightmare.

I was born in Bulawayo, Rhodesia and moved to the UK in 2008. I have worked in the Police since 2011.

My childhood was a mixed bag. On one hand it was deeply filled with trauma that would mess up any child and on the other hand it contained some beautiful memories. I was sexually abused at a very young age by multiple men. I was physically abused to extents which make me cringe with disgust now. The emotional abuse was an ongoing thing. I have only just been able to speak out about the abuse recently, forty years later.

My childhood was not all bad, I grew up riding bikes, fishing, playing in the mud etc. My parents were divorced and the difference between the two houses were like chalk and cheese. When everything got too much my brother and I asked my dad if we could move in with him and we went from a life of having to make our own meals from a very early age to a stable environment. Unfortunately, the damage had been done by then and I wasn't to know that until I got older, and pain plagued my body.

When I was 19, I met Trevor, my husband, and we got married when I was 20. We had two beautiful daughters who are the light of our lives and then I found out I was pregnant with a son.

We were beyond excited as having a little boy completed our family. The pregnancy was going well apart from the fact that Tyler was not growing as fast as he should have. We went to see specialists in Harare (275 miles ish) every month to have the baby monitored and he seemed to be doing everything right. It was decided that I would have the baby in Harare to ensure that the medical team was on hand. The day of the c section arrived, and we were beyond excited. I went into surgery and shortly afterwards Tyler was born. I went back to my ward and assumed that the baby was not brought to me as I had just had surgery and needed to recover.

That evening the paediatric cardiologist visited me and told me that my son had a heart murmur and after tests the following day it was confirmed that he had Hyperplastic Left Heart Syndrome. We were told that we had to fly our son to South Africa for a series of three operations to basically rebuild his heart. These operations would give Tyler a 10% chance of life. If he did not receive the operations, he would sadly pass away within the next three days. We made the decision to do everything we could for Tyler and with financial help from family and friends flew him to South Africa where his little heart was operated on. The operation went well, and Tyler came out fighting. He was such a strong little boy and brought so much light into all our lives. Unfortunately, at three months old he went into cardiac arrest and passed away.

There is a lot more to this story and I will post links at the end if you want to read it. It proves that miracles are everywhere and do happen.

A month after Tyler passed away, I found out that I was pregnant. I was petrified. I never wanted to go through the heartbreak of losing another baby. Every check-up, every movement, every pain had me worrying that something was wrong. Those nine months were the longest nine months of my life, and I spent them worrying non-stop. However, on the 6th October 2004 I went into surgery and came out with a beautiful, healthy baby boy. I took one look at this gorgeous baby and my heart melted; my family was complete.

Charmaine II

After the birth, I found myself aching more than normal. I put it down to having kids, after all I had done this four times now. I carried on being a mother and wife and loving every minute of it however I still had this fear of something going wrong.

With the crime and healthcare in Zimbabwe being pretty scary my husband and I made the decision to move to the UK so that if anything should happen to our children at least we could get them into a hospital. We applied for our ancestry visas. We sold everything we had but unfortunately Robert Mugabe's ruling was that you could not take foreign currency out of the country. We managed to stuff six hundred pounds into our shoes and clothing, packed a suitcase of belongings each and took the long flight to Cheshire, UK. One of the restrictions on our visas was the fact that we were not entitled to any public funds so once we arrived here it was a case of work or be destitute.

Trev went out to work packing vegetables at first which was hard on him and the family after he was a branch manager in Zimbabwe. It caused a lot of stress on the family and eventually he got a job as a vehicle mechanic. Whilst all this was going on my aches and pains carried on and I put it down to stress.

I had several doctors' appointments over the years and got told the same thing, "You are overweight". Of course, I am overweight, I can't move.

Fast forward to 2017, we were settled, and things were going well albeit the pain. My Mom had had various cancer scares over the last few years, and I was travelling between Cheshire and Huddersfield frequently to take her to doctors' appointments.

My pain was by now really bad, and I spent every moment I could in bed. Every time I saw a doctor, they put me on more painkillers. I pushed myself to keep doing my chores, looking after Mom, working and being a mother and wife but things were becoming difficult. I went to my GP in tears and told him I can't carry on. I was well and truly broken. He did the various tests which had me sobbing uncontrollably with the pain when he finally diagnosed me with Fibromyalgia. This relief filled my body. I finally knew what was causing the pain and we could fix it. The doctor prescribed me amitriptyline, gabapentine, codeine and sertraline and told me to see him in a couple of weeks' time. I went home and took this cocktail of pills and went to sleep. I slept for eighteen hours straight and woke up and shortly after went back to sleep. Little did I know but this was the start of my troubles.

By now, Mom was diagnosed with sclc (small cell lung cancer) and was given six months to live. I didn't want to let her down so the only time I dragged myself out of bed was to take her to doctors' appointments. I wasn't much help as I could not think properly, couldn't remember anything. I was a wreck. I went back to the doctor who added naproxen and a sleeping tablet to the mix. I would wake up in the morning and try to concentrate on my work which was impossible. My boss could not understand what brain fog was and was doubting the effects of the Fibro and the huge cocktail of pills. Mom passed away in 2019 and I came home and went to bed.

I started drinking wine at night to help me sleep and to take away the pain. It started with one bottle a night (that is only three glasses, right?) and by the middle of 2022 I was having a minimum of two bottles, sometimes three bottles of wine a night. By now I did not get out of bed other than to use the toilet and bath. I wanted life to end. I could not take it anymore.

A colleague and now very good friend, Mike Denton had organised an online session with various speakers for Fibromyalgia Day at work. I was curious and thought I can't lose anything by watching it. A consultant specialising in Fibromyalgia was speaking about a new trial coming up to prove that Fibromyalgia could be diagnosed in the blood. For anyone who knows how long it takes to get a Fibro diagnosis this could be incredible news. Another lady called Jules Kelly (soon to be my fairy godmother) spoke about the The Life Freedom Method® which incorporated numerous modalities. As soon as I heard Jules speak, I felt excited. She was speaking my language. Jules did not agree with shovelling pills down patient's throats and was more interested in healing the trauma inside which in turn heals the physical pain. I could not get enough of what she was saying. This truly resonated with me, and I commented on everything she said just to get noticed.

A couple of weeks later, Mike contacted me to let me know that the trial was being opened to a few people in Cheshire Police to check whether we had the Fibro antibodies in our blood. I jumped at the chance to be tested. How cool would it be to be one of the first people to be properly tested for Fibromyalgia. Little did I know that this was only the beginning and what seemed like such a massive step forward in medical science was only the tip of the iceberg. Jules Kelly was about to change my entire life.

Charmaine III

Jules had offered to go one step further and offer Mike and I twelve weeks of her time to improve try and help us Fibromyalgia. I was ecstatic. Everything this lady said resonated with me and I was so ready to try anything to get better.

Mike and I went to the Walton Centre in Liverpool to have our bloods taken. Eight big vials of blood were taken, and pressure tests were done. The pressure tests were so painful. As soon as the doctor pressed anywhere the pain was excruciating. A sensitivity test was then done where our arms were stroked continuously. The sensation lasted the entire day and I have never been so uncomfortable. Both Mike and I were re-diagnosed with Fibromyalgia and classed as disabled. I felt so disappointed in myself and was telling myself how stupid and weak I was.

The big day with Jules arrived and I went to the meeting with my diet coke. I drank up to three litres of diet coke a day at the time. As soon as Jules saw it, she smiled. She knew how much our lives were about to change.

Mike and I had been chatting about what to expect with these sessions and we were convinced Jules was going to make us drink camel pee and do goat yoga. Luckily, she only made us commit to drinking two litres of water a day, take some supplements and journal our thoughts, feelings, symptoms etc. During the session Jules shared the plant / Fanta analogy with us and showed us how if you water a plant, give it sunshine and nutrients it will thrive. If you however give it Fanta and keep it in a dark place it will get sick and die. After the session I went back to my desk, put the diet coke down and have never had another sip of it.

During the following sessions Jules gave us an overview of essential oils, created natural morphine bombs (lemongrass, oregano, frankincense, marjoram) which are incredible, and introduced us to doTERRA Deep Blue. The Deep Blue was my saving grace. Anytime I felt pain I rubbed this magic stuff on, and the pain went. It was amazing and the best part is that it is completely natural. Initially, I used it every time I had pain but after processing the trauma which caused the pain, I haven't used it in months.

I have cut out all medications apart from my sertraline and blood pressure medication. I do advise you to speak to your doctor before doing this. I had no issues, but everyone is different.

Up until this moment I had been doing EMDR for about two years. I have had eighty sessions altogether. It had certainly helped me deal with some of the trauma, but it hadn't touched the pain.

During my sessions with Jules, she taught me The Human Compass® which is a way in which your subconscious answers questions using your body without you thinking about them. We used this to determine trapped emotions which were causing the body to put out pain, the age of the trauma, things the mind had blocked out to protect us.

Jules introduced us to Human Design which is explained in the Life Freedom Method®. Human Design teaches you how to live to the best of your ability. It shows you your strengths and weaknesses and teaches you how to enhance your life. Human Design helped me understand my family better and why they do the things they do. My children and I used to clash constantly because as soon as they did anything wrong, I would chastise them. Through learning this framework, I have learnt to step back, take a deep breath and once everyone has calmed down to speak to the children rather than at them. Embodying the learnings of Human Design has brought calmness and understanding into my house. My son, however, tends to use it against me by telling me he is a thinker not a doer so should not be made to do things. Clever, huh!!!

Jules' business partner, Claire, took Mike and I through a fourteen-day meditation course which we can use whenever things get a bit crazy. I feel like it has given me the grounding and the peace in my life that I desperately needed. The meditation has taught me how to use my breath to calm myself. It has improved my sleep pattern and gives me the energy when I need it depending on the meditation.

If you aren't into woo woo stuff stop reading now!!!!!!! You will, however, never know the secret of how to change the limiting beliefs which keep the trauma trapped in our bodies resulting in pain.

So, as I explained before, I have a lot of traumas to sort out. Jules was able to help me process all this trauma using Belief Coding®, a modality which was created by Jessica Cunningham. The Belief Coding® technique helps to remove the emotional charge from a

31

past traumatic experience response, to allowing the patient to live free from pain by resolving the cellular memory of that trauma response experience.

My way of explaining Belief Coding® is with a car analogy. Before I processed the trauma, I would think of what happened and felt like a car came crashing into me each time. It was terrifying. After processing the trauma, I feel like the car still comes towards me when I think about it, but it carries on by calmly. This is because it has removed the emotional charge from the trauma.

Since working with Jules, I have cleared all my trauma and subsequently my pain in eight sessions. I am now able to identify why my body is putting out pain and just by understanding what my body is trying to tell me I can clear any trapped emotions and therefore clear the pain. After my sessions with Jules, I was able to go with Mike to one of Jessica's in person training seminars and am currently working towards becoming accredited as a Belief Coding® facilitator.

My mind has been opened to so many possibilities. I am learning new skills and whereas before I wanted my life to be over, I am excited about life now. I remember stuff I learn. I have this clarity that is quite overwhelming at times. I love learning how to help others and cannot get enough of it.

Before my twelve weeks with Jules, family outings always ended up with me being miserable as I was always tired and always in pain. In order to try fix myself I drank wine which brought out an angry side to me. I was angry that I was hurting, angry that I was tired, angry that I was missing out on life.

I have been able to cut out alcohol during the week and cut right down on weekends. The next step of my journey is to cut out alcohol all together and I am excited about that.

Since clearing my traumas my children want to be around me and go for family outings. A few weeks ago, we went to the zoo together and I walked fifteen thousand steps. I came home dreading the following day as I was so used to being sore after exercise. The following day I woke up and apart from a little stiffness I felt absolutely fine. After so many years of feeling so broken it takes a while to accept that actually you are great. I keep waiting for the other shoe to drop and am slowly but surely accepting that there is no other shoe. Once the trauma is cleared, that is it. There is no pain. Absolutely everything in life is made up of energy and by turning that negative energy into positive energy you can get through anything and everything.

I have always loved gardening, however, for so long I have been in too much pain to do any. This year my garden is full of beautiful flowers. Every time I look outside at my flowers I am filled with happiness and am in awe that I did all of that. It sounds a bit weird, but I feel as though I have been reborn, like the world is clearer and more beautiful than ever before.

After our twelve weeks with Jules, Mike and I went back to the Walton centre and all the tests were redone. The pressure tests did not affect us at all, the sensitivity test was a walk in the park and at the end of the session the doctor had nothing else to say other than, "You no longer meet the criteria to be classed as disabled". How incredible is that?

My future looks very bright due to three beautiful ladies and their modalities. I plan on being accredited very soon and start helping others to get over the trauma that has been holding them back, to give them their lives back.

I plan to carry on with my studies and to learn everything I can to be able to give back the beauty in life to those who are suffering. I plan to spend loads more time with my husband of twenty-five years now and my beautiful children and their partners and eventually my grandbabies. Life is exciting and wonderful.

I want to thank you for taking the time to read my story. I hope it shows you that there is always a light at the end of the tunnel and that light is so bright and beautiful. None of my healing has been impossibly hard. Some parts of it have not exactly been a walk in the park but when you come out the other side and you feel incredible, and your pain is gone it is so worth it. There is absolutely no reason why anyone should live feeling despondent and in pain.

Your new life is here. You just need to reach out and grab it.

Charmaine.

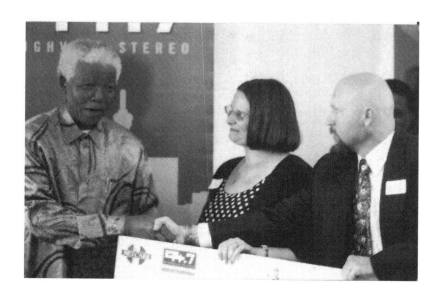

This is a picture of my husband Trevor and myself handing over the cheque for one million rand which was raised for Tyler's treatment. When Tyler passed, we donated the money to the Walter Sisulu fund to enable other children with heart problems to get the treatment they normally would not be able to afford.

Below is the Tree of Life which was painted in the hospital as a legacy to Tyler. Each leaf on the tree represents a child who was treated through the fund for Tyler. there was a new sense of purpose in her step as she set off.

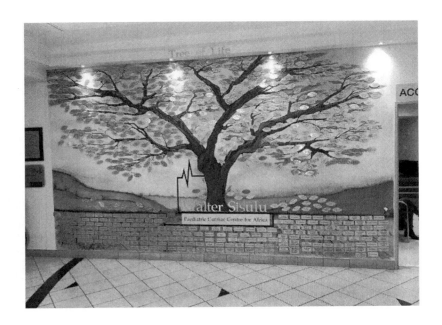

Jules, Claire & Jessica

"Purpose"

Definition:

The reason for which something is done or created or for which something exists.

"the purpose of the meeting is to appoint a trustee."

a person's sense of resolve or determination.

"there was a new sense of purpose in her step as she set off.""

The twelve weeks that Mike, Charmaine, Claire, Jessica and I spent together was full of purpose.

Twelve weeks spent in the company of these two incredible individuals has reaffirmed to us that The Life Freedom Method® is one of the main ways in which we are to deliver our purpose in this lifetime. We are here to help people live without pain and to understand that they have one life and always two choices.

Mike and Charmaine have shown that they had a resounding purpose to get well, and they now have a whole new sense of purpose as they continue to share their journey and their message.

The results speak for themselves. You only need to look at them both to know that they are in a whole new world now. The medical results for those that need them merely confirm what we already knew.

The "system" requires unequivocal proof that The Life Freedom

Method® works to enable it to be offered to all. We aim to do this by way of further research and randomised clinical trial.

Our vision and drive is to bring The Life Freedom Method® as a recognised solution to Chronic Pain and Fibromyalgia to the mainstream, available to all.

We know that we are pioneering change in performance via holistic science backed wellbeing practices. We understand that this is not something yet widely acknowledged or understood. We understand that there are people that will not understand or want to understand the work that we are doing. We also understand that the route to making this approach readily available will not be a walk in the park.

We do however strongly believe that it is so needed in our society today and we will continue to share our journey with anyone that wishes to be a part of it.

The initial pilot with Mike and Charmaine was accompanied by a white paper that we presented to the medics to understand the scientific underpinning of each step of The Life Freedom Method®.

This is shared with you here, followed by the laboratory results from the NHS Walton Centre and Liverpool University.

We are extremely grateful for the opportunity Dr Goebel and his team gave to us and all their cooperation to allow us to trial our Life Freedom Method® in its earliest days.

Thanks to you for reading our story.

Jules,Claire & Jessica

Fibromyalgia Trauma Patient Report _ Mike

Thank you so much for participating in our study.

Clinical Examination
Following examination, on your first visit, you met the criteria for Fibromyalgia Syndrome (American College of Rheumatology 2010). On your second visit, you did not. It is important to say that there is little research to describe what happens to patients on a day-to-day basis, and symptom fluctuation is a normal part of the disorder, however, your symptoms were objectively much improved.

Individual tests

Questionnaire (out of)	Before	After	Improved?	Meaning
Widespread Pain Index (19)	15	6		Pain distribution receded
Symptom Severity Score (12)	8	2		Symptoms such as fatigue, sleep, cognitive and general somatic problems improved
Tender Points (19)	6	2		Less deep tenderness
Arm Pressure Pain Threshold (kPa)	169	271.7		Able to tolerate a higher skin pressure over arms
Leg Pressure Pain Threshold (kPa)	426.7	726.7		Able to withstand a higher skin pressure over legs
Slow stroke Pleasantness (-5 to 5)	2	5		Enjoy stroking much more
Fast stroke Pleasantness (-5 to 5)	2.3	5		Enjoy stroking much more
After Sensations	YES	N		Less likely to receive strange sensations after touch
Pain Level (10)	6	1		Less pain
EQ5D (25)	9	7		Improved Quality of life
Health Rating	50	89.5		Improved self-health rating out of 100
Brief Pain Index (70)	19	1		Much improved impact of pain on activities of daily living
Hospital Anxiety Score (21)	12	4		Much less anxiety
Hospital Depression Score (21)	8	7		Similar depression but below cut off used or 8/21
Pain Catastrophising Score (52)	18	5		Less likely to think the worst related to your pain but both below the clinically relevant cut off.
Patient Self Efficacy Score (60)	32	55		More able to manage your pain on your own
Fibromyalgia Impact Questionnaire (100)	40.8	19.5		Much improved impact of fibromyalgia symptoms on your life
Pain DETECT (38)	20	8		Less neuropathic (nerve like) pain
Fatigue (10)	5	3		More energy

The Antibody Test

Antibodies are immune proteins found in the body which stick to pathogens (bugs). They earmark these pathogens for destruction by other parts of the immune system. They can cause auto-immune disease if there is a fault in the production of them, and they stick to the cells of the body, rather than pathogens. These are called self or (auto)antibodies. The stickiness of antibodies can be very important, and they are usually very specific to the target protein to which they were developed. Our result suggested that autoantibodies may be involved in some cases of fibromyalgia.

The way we test for these self-directed, autoantibodies is to prepare some special cells we think are particularly important in fibromyalgia. These are called satellite glial cells which are support cells for nerves. They are part of the peripheral nervous system (the part of the body which senses pain, which is not the brain or spinal cord). We treat these cells with a purified mixture of all the long-lasting (memory) antibodies found in your blood. We wash these cells to leave the antibodies that stick very strongly. These remaining antibodies are autoantibodies. We then test the amount of autoantibody with a fluorescent dye which reports how much of these autoantibodies have stuck to the satellite glial cells.

Your Results
The antibody tests suggested that **the level of these antibodies in your blood was low which was checked twice. There was no significant difference at follow up.**

We know that there is variation in the amount of these antibodies present in patients (please see link below by one of our collaborators). Also, it is likely that the condition of fibromyalgia may not just be produced by one way.

https://journals.lww.com/pain/Fulltext/9900/Fibromyalgia_patients_with_elevated_levels_of.274.aspx

We are so very pleased that the trauma treatment has worked for you and as is clear from the results it has very much improved your symptoms.

R Berwick 2023

41

Fibromyalgia Trauma Patient Report _ Charmaine

Thank you so much for participating in our study.

Following examination, on your first visit, you met the criteria for Fibromyalgia Syndrome (American College of Rheumatology 2010). On your second visit, you did not. It is important to say that there is little research to describe what happens to patients on a day-to-day basis, and symptom fluctuation is a normal part of the disorder, however, your symptoms were objectively much improved.

Individual tests

Questionnaire (out of)	Before	After	Improved?	Meaning
Widespread Pain Index (19)	18	1		Pain greatly distribution receded
Symptom Severity Score (12)	9	5		Symptoms such as fatigue, sleep, cognitive and general somatic problems improved
Tender Points (19)	16	8		Less deep tenderness
Arm Pressure Pain Threshold (kPa)	110	213.3		Able to tolerate a higher skin pressure over arms
Leg Pressure Pain Threshold (kPa)	123.4	453.3		Able to withstand a higher skin pressure over legs
Slow stroke Pleasantness (-5 to 5)	-3	0		Can stand stroking much more, used to be very unpleasant now neither pleasant or unpleasant.
Fast stroke Pleasantness (-5 to 5)	—1	0.7		Enjoy stroking much more, used to be very unpleasant.
After Sensations	YES	No		Less likely to receive strange unpleasant sensations after touch
Pain Level (10)	8	0		Less pain
EQ5D (25)	13	6		Improved Quality of life
Health Rating	75	90		Improved self-health rating out of 100
Brief Pain Index (70)	54	2		Much improved impact of pain on activities of daily living
Hospital Anxiety Score (21)	13	3		Much less anxiety
Hospital Depression Score (21)	7	3		Similar depression but below cut off
Pain Catastrophising Score (52)	19	1		Less likely to think the worst related to your pain but both below the clinically relevant cut off.
Patient Self Efficacy Score (60)	22	60		Much more able to manage your pain on your own
Fibromyalgia Impact Questionnaire (100)	74.7	14.3		Much improved impact of fibromyalgia symptoms on your life
Pain DETECT (38)	22	6		Less neuropathic (nerve like) pain
Fatigue (10)	10	1		So much more energy

The Antibody Test

R Berwick 2023

Antibodies are immune proteins found in the body which stick to pathogens (bugs). They earmark these pathogens for destruction by other parts of the immune system. They can cause auto-immune disease if there is a fault in the production of them, and they stick to the cells of the body, rather than pathogens. These are called self or (auto)antibodies. The stickiness of antibodies can be very important, and they are usually very specific to the target protein to which they were developed. Our result suggested that autoantibodies may be involved in some cases of fibromyalgia.

The way we test for these self-directed, autoantibodies is to prepare some special cells we think are particularly important in fibromyalgia. These are called satellite glial cells which are support cells for nerves. They are part of the peripheral nervous system (the part of the body which senses pain, which is not the brain or spinal cord). We treat these cells with a purified mixture of all the long-lasting (memory) antibodies found in your blood. We wash these cells to leave the antibodies that stick very strongly. These remaining antibodies are autoantibodies. We then test the amount of autoantibody with a fluorescent dye which reports how much of these autoantibodies have stuck to the satellite glial cells.

Your Results
The antibody tests suggested that **the level of these antibodies in your blood was low which was checked twice. There was no significant difference at follow up compared to before .**

We know that there is variation in the amount of these antibodies present in patients (please see link below by one of our collaborators). Also, it is likely that the condition of fibromyalgia may not just be produced by one way.

https://journals.lww.com/pain/Fulltext/9900/Fibromyalgia_patients_with_elevated_levels_of.274.aspx

We are so very pleased that the trauma treatment has worked for you and as is clear from the results it has very much improved your symptoms.

R Berwick 2023

43

We are delighted with our results and to have had this opportunity been part of the start of this pioneering movement of change.

We hope that our journey inspires you in some small way.

Mike & Charmaine

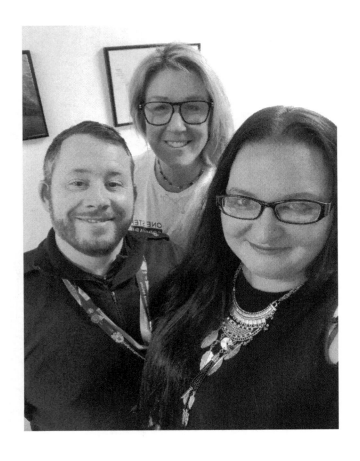

This is us with Jules Kelly at Cheshire Police HQ on the final day of our 12-week Life Freedom Method® Programme before we went to have our final tests with the medics at the Walton Centre, Liverpool.

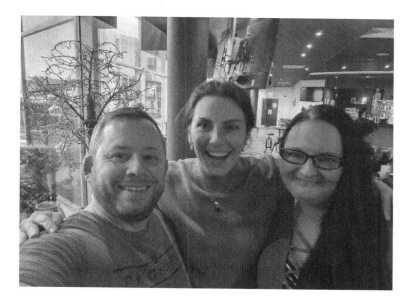

This is us with Jessica Cunningham at the Belief Coding® Facilitator Training in Sheffield.

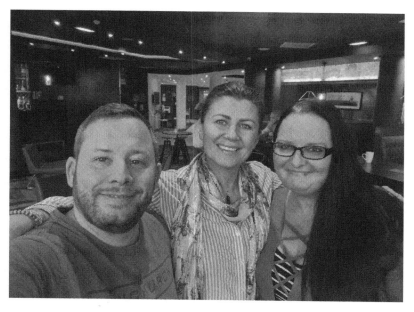

This is us with Claire Morton at the in person Belief Coding® Facilitator Training in Sheffield.

If we have inspired you and you would like us to come and speak at one of your events to share our story then please contact us at

char@disabledtoenabled@gmail.com

mike@disabledtoenabled@gmail.com

To find out more about The Life Freedom Method® and to contact Jules Kelly, Claire Morton & Jessica Cunningham, you can find them at www.spaceandfreedom.com

To find out more about the natural essential oils and supplements that we used during the trial then Charmaine would be happy to help.

Char@disabledtoenabled@gmail.com

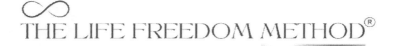

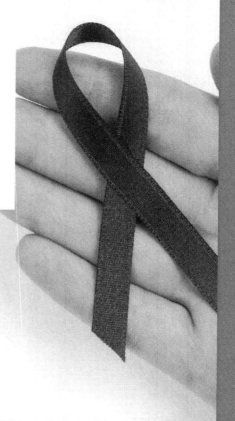

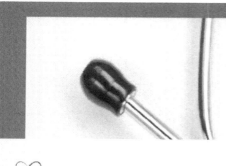

THE LIFE FREEDOM METHOD®

EVIDENCE
SYNTHESIS

PREPARED BY
JULES KELLY
Space and Freedom Limited

REVIEWED BY
PROFESSOR BEN KELLY
Professor of Population & Clinical
Data Science
Nuffield Health & Manchester
Metropolitan University

Introduction

Fibromyalgia is a chronic pain condition affecting more than 2 million people in the UK and 2-4% of the US population, characterised by widespread pain, fatigue and brain fog.

The diagnosis of Fibromyalgia can be challenging; there are no known clinical laboratory investigations to confirm or refute its presence. Symptoms are commonly multiple, can fluctuate and may not easily sit within established medical diagnostic categories. It can often be difficult for patients to articulate their array of symptoms, and for both patients and healthcare professionals to fully make sense of the complexities of the condition. Due to these factors, patients may be diagnosed inaccurately with alternative conditions; only receive a Fibromyalgia diagnosis after years of delay, or sometimes be inaccurately diagnosed with Fibromyalgia. Living with the symptoms of the condition can fundamentally impact on a person's quality of life.

Treatment options available in the UK are limited to exercise in various forms, talking therapies, such as Cognitive Behavioural Therapy (CBT) and Acceptance and Commitment therapy (ACT) as well as pharmacological therapies such as Antidepressants including Amitriptyline, Citalopram, Duloxetine, Fluoxetine and Sertraline. Drugs such as Gabapentin, (Neurontin) Pregabalin (Lyrica) and Codeine are also regularly prescribed. Each of these drugs has their own side effects that can also impact the patient's wellbeing and quality of life and in the main, the patient continues to live with a level of chronic pain. There is little information on option s of pain removal, with pain management being the primary focus of most available treatment options. The International Classification of Diseases most recent iteration (ICD-11) includes fibromyalgia as a 'third level diagnoses' under the grouping MG3 0.01 - chronic widespread pain, which is a subgroup of chronic primary pain.

Recent research has revealed important evidence for changes in central and peripheral nervous system functions and immunological activity. Dr Andreas Goebel and his team at The Walton Centre, Liverpool have carried out a breakthrough study, that demonstrates that Fibromyalgia may be a disease of the immune system, which could transform how the condition is viewed and help to lead to new and improved treatments.1 Further work is required to evaluate new treatment regimens that could be standalone or complimentary.

Background

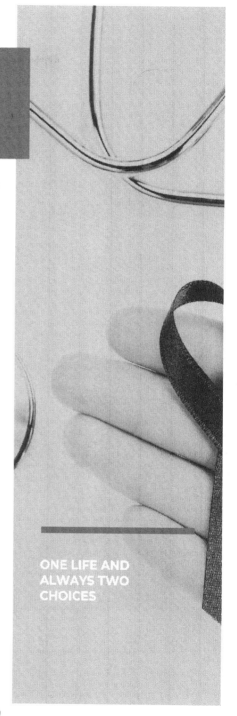

Jules Kelly was invited to carry out a pilot study of the Life Freedom Method® as part of the work of Dr Andreas Goebel and his team. The pilot involved introducing 3 patients to the Liverpool University APIF Study. 2 They were accepted after having been examined and blood samples taken to explore the role of the immune system and specific antibodies present in people living with Fibromyalgia. They were then passed back to work with Jules Kelly to work with The Life Freedom Method®. The work was carried out over a period of 12 weeks

Objectives

The objectives of the pilot work are four-fold:

- To reduce subjective pain from the body as measured by the Brief Pain Inventory (Short For), and the pressure tests carried out by the APIF Team at the Walton Centre.
- To improve Quality of Life as measured by the EQ-5D-5L.
- To demonstrate a link between the completion of the Life Freedom Method® and a change in the binding of antibodies to the cells in the Dorsal Root Ganglia activity
- To publish pilot data with the intent to use findings as a foundation for RCT funding application.

ONE LIFE AND
ALWAYS TWO
CHOICES

49

Methods & Aims

THIS DESKTOP SYSTEMATIC ANALYSIS OF THE LITERATURE WAS COMPLETED TO ESTABLISH THE POTENTIAL MECHANISTIC UNDER PINNINGS THAT MAY INFLUENCE PAIN MANAGEMENT WITH SPECIFIC APPLICATION TO THE LIFE FREEDOM METHOD®.

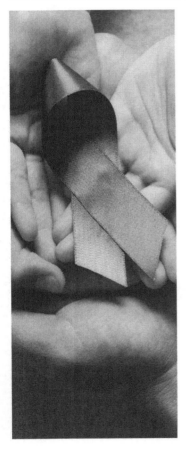

The Key elements of the Life Freedom Method® are a combination of the following:

- Wellbeing education

- Nutrition

- Hydration

- Aromatherapy

- Positive Psychology and Belief

- Management

- Meditation

- Journaling

- Coaching

- Trauma Work - Belief Coding®

- Energy Healing

Whilst each individual component has evidence to underpin its effectiveness, the challenge remains that there may be no current theoretically underpinned for all of the interventions being deployed together to reach the desired outcomes.

Aims

The primary aim of the pilot activity is to investigate the impact of The Life Freedom Method® on antibody concentrations related to Dorsal Root Ganglia activity and quality of life in those living with Fibromyalgia.

∞
THE LIFE FREEDOM METHOD®

STEP 1

Those entering the programme enter into a verbal contract agreement. This consists of:

a. Confirming that they are ready to become well.

b. Confirming that they will follow the recommendations of the LFM and as lead by the facilitator.

c. Confirming their commitment to doing anything that is required to enable their body to heal.

d. Confirming that their body and their health and wellbeing is their own overall responsibility.

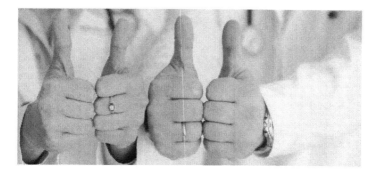

STEP 2

Positive consultation and sharing is a key initial process within the programme. It has been demonstrated that positive consultation[2] and sharing is a way to significantly reduce pain. This coupled with the fact that the subjects have taken an intentional step to wellness to gain access to this pilot trial also supports their dedicated invested position in the process.

STEP 3

Building a relationship and understanding of the subjects, their challenges and life circumstances alongside the process is a critical early step. As is having an open, empathetic and honest relationship between the facilitator and the subject helps to build trust quickly. It has been demonstrated that empathy lowers patients' anxiety and distress and is of unquestionable importance.[3]

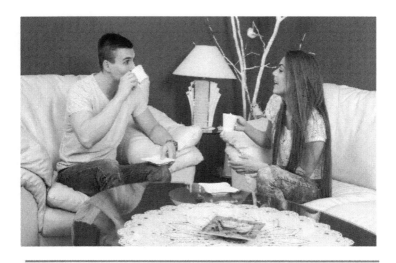

STEP 4

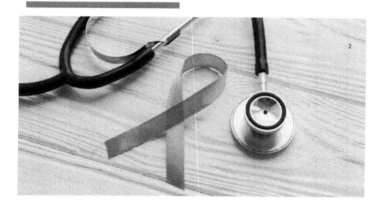

Introducing a level of belief in the subjects that they can and will feel better in just a few weeks' time plays an important role in the process.

Removing the common blocks for procrastination; self-sabotage; and non-starting (financial burden) are all tools utilised within the process. This is achieved through the use of coaching and using the Belief Coding® technique (full details within section 10)

It has been demonstrated that belief plays a major role in the recovery of the subject. If subjects expect that they will feel a reduction in pain, this expectation causes their brain to produce its own painkiller by the release of substantial amounts of endogenous dopamine in both the dorsal and ventral striatum, which then reduces the experience of pain. It may be suggested that 'belief' mirrors what would be classified in RCT's as placebo. Harnessing the placebo effect has been demonstrated many times.

Fabrizio Benedetti, Professor of Physiology and Neuroscience at the University of Turin Medical School demonstrated this effect in a study involving Parkinson's disease patients. They showed that the placebo created a change in physical biochemistry. A strong positive response has been demonstrated using a placebo in the reduction of pain and other symptoms in people living with Fibromyagia.[6]

STEP 5

The Life Freedom Method® takes a holistic approach to therapy, looking at the body, mind and lifestyle when working to address pain. Education is provided on human physiology, including nutrition; toxic load and its impact; trauma education provides a basic grounding to enable subjects to visualise what is being subjectively experienced and the potential influence lifestyle choices have on overall pain and wellbeing.

Subjects are given a face-to- face overview session and a 15 module programme that provides basic information on the benefits of keeping the body hydrated; reducing their toxic load; nutrition; the impact of stress and anxiety on the body; the impact of overall wellbeing through understanding lifestyle choices and their impact on the body's endocrine system; understanding metabolism and how maximise energy levels; how to support the immune system; aromatherapy and meditation.

A recent meta-analysis confirms education can lead to more considered choices that lead to better health. [7]

Furthermore, studies have demonstrated that computer based programs for people with chronic disease may combine health information with online peer support, decision support, or help with behaviour change. Such programs have been shown to increase knowledge, feelings of social support, and some clinical outcomes among users [8]

Computer-based programs can also be useful for behavioural risk reduction in areas such as smoking and diet. [9]

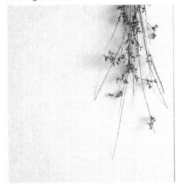

STEP 6

Step 6 is a comprehensive nutritional intervention. Water intake and Nutrition is the grounding for supporting the cellular health of the body.

Alongside the education piece, the subjects are provided with fully bio available nutritional supplementation and a directive to drink a minimum of 2 litres of water per day. Whilst having overall wellness benefits it has been documented by Field et al that diet, its quality and its nutritional density may be involved in modulating pain physiology.[10]Whilst the main question of this document is around reduction of pain, there is also evidence that water intake has a positive impact on another key challenge observed by Fibromyalgia patients, Brain Fog.[11]

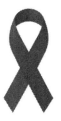

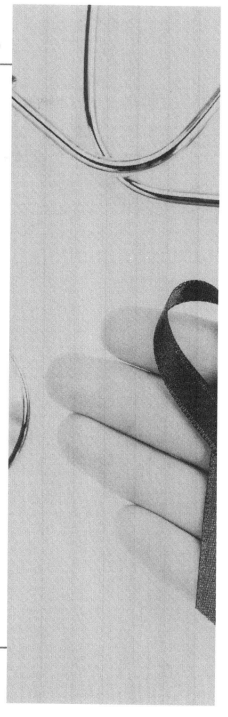

55

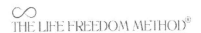

NUTRITIONAL DETAIL

Developing chronic musculoskeletal pain may be driven by mechanisms beyond traditional psychological and cognitive systems to which it is often attributed. In fact, the WHO suggests the diet support modulation of pain in the body and recognises its importance as a "modifiable determinant" of pain. For example, eicosapentaenoic acids, arachidonic acids, and tryptophan, all of which are essential fatty acids, have been linked in producing pain-relieving effects at the CNS level.[12]

Nutrient supplementation is a broadly investigated treatment modality as numerous nutrient and vitamin deficiencies have been linked to Fibromyalgia and whilst preliminary results are promising, much of the existing evidence regarding diet supplementation is of poor quality. Further robust studies are needed to fully elucidate the potential of this complimentary therapeutic option.[13]

Within the Life Freedom Method®, subjects were each provided with a 4- month supply of a high quality bioavailable nutritional supplementation. The manufacturer has run their own clinical trials with these supplements, with results showing statistically significant improvement after supplementation: blood lipids, fasting insulin, cardiovascular biomarkers, EPA, and the AA/EPA ratio. These health biomarkers showed that the" Lifelong Vitality Pack" supplements had positive effects on biochemical indicators of cardiovascular health, antioxidant status, inflammation levels, and blood glucose regulation.

Subjects reported more mental clarity, energy, motivation, control, balance, happiness, and several subjective measures of health improvement after taking the supplements consistently for two months, as measured by dōTERRA. The results provide scientific substantiation that these supplements taken alongside the daily diet may support cardiovascular health, metabolic health, inflammation status, antioxidant status, energy level, immunity, and mood.

Full report details have been requested however in the interim, the details of the contents and the theoretical underpinning of the contents are as follows: -

XEO OMEGA
INGREDIENTS

xEO Mega Essential Oil Omega complex (Doterra, USA) is a unique formula of Certified Pure Tested Grade™ essential oils and a proprietary blend of marine and plant sourced omega fatty acids. One serving of xEO Mega provides 450 mg of marine lipids (providing 150 mg of EPA, 150 mg of DHA, and 30 mg of other omega 3s), and a blend of 125 mg of plant-sourced fatty acids. xEO Mega also includes 10 mcg of natural vitamin D, 20 mg of natural vitamin E, and .5 mg of astaxanthin, an antioxidant carotenoid harvested from microalgae.[5]

These fatty acids are able to partly inhibit a number of aspects of inflammation including leukocyte chemotaxis, adhesion molecule expression and leukocyte-endothelial adhesive interactions, production of eicosanoids like prostaglandins and leukotrienes from the n-6 fatty acid arachidonic acid, production of inflammatory cytokines, and T- helper 1 lymphocyte reactivity. In addition, EPA gives rise to eicosanoids that often have lower biological potency than those produced from arachidonic acid and EPA and DHA give rise to anti-inflammatory and inflammation resolving mediators called resolvins, protectins and maresins. [15]

ALA and SDA xEO Mega delivers a unique source of plant-based oils derived from the Ahiflower (Buglossoides arvensis). Cold-pressed Ahiflower seed oil provides a concentrated source of both ALA and SDA, which the body can convert more easily to EPA. Both ALA and SDA promote cardiovascular health.

ALA and SDA are produced by many plants, but because of the low number of vegetables consumed in the standard Western diet, they are often not consumed in adequate amounts. "food staples and food processing procedures introduced during the Neolithic and Industrial Periods have fundamentally altered 7 crucial nutritional characteristics of ancestral hominin diets: 1) glycemic load, 2) fatty acid composition, 3) macronutrient composition, 4) micronutrient density, 5) acid-base balance, 6) sodium-potassium ratio, and 7) fibre content. The evolutionary collision of our ancient genome with the nutritional qualities of recently introduced foods may underlie many of the chronic diseases of Western civilization."[14]

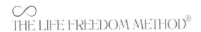
XEO OMEGA
INGREDIENTS

Ahiflower seed oil also delivers GLA, which may help support the health of joints, lungs, and the nervous system. Strong support exists for gamma linolenic acid (GLA) for pain of rheumatoid arthritis (RA)[16]and recent research has identified several new mechanisms of action that help to explain previously identified effects of n-3 fatty acids on inflammation and immunity. Astaxanthin[17] and Vitamin E Omega-3 fatty acids are important for circulatory and brain health. The brain is made up of essential lipids that, as with the free lipids traveling in the circulatory system, are prone to degradation through free-radical oxidation. xEO Mega includes the powerful antioxidant carotenoid astaxanthin that helps protect against lipid oxidation in the brain and throughout the circulatory system. Astaxanthin provides powerful antioxidant and circulatory benefits, supports eye health, improves muscle strength and endurance, aids the liver and digestive system, supports skin health, and promotes healthy immune function. The astaxanthin used in xEO Mega is a standardized extract of microalgae cultivated in a pure water system and activated by light. In response to exposure to light, the microalgae produces astaxanthin as a defence mechanism against oxidation. The microalgae changes from a light green to a deep crimson red. The astaxanthin is then extracted from the microalgae, microfiltered, and standardized for potency. The astaxanthin is coupled with natural vitamin E to provide additional circulatory and systemic benefits as powerful antioxidant additions to the antioxidant essential oils in xEO Mega ®.

xEO Mega also includes 10 mcg of natural vitamin D. Vitamin D is a fatsoluble vitamin present in a limited number of foods such as fish, beef liver, cheese, egg yolks, and fortified dairy products. It can also be synthesized in the body when triggered by exposure to sunlight. Vitamin D plays an essential role in bone health and growth. As with the omega-3 fatty acids in xEO Mega®, vitamin D also plays an important role in promoting healthy immune function and a healthy response to oxidative stress.

Studies suggest a possible role of vitamin D supplementation in alleviating the pain associated with Fibromyalgia, especially in vitamin D-deficient individuals.[18]

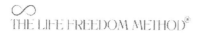

THE LIFE FREEDOM METHOD®

OTHER KEY INGREDIENTS

Some other key ingredients to the supplementation that support the body by way of reduction in pain or overall wellbeing have been included with supporting underpinning information.

CLOVE ESSENTIAL OIL

Clove Oil (Eugenia carophyllata, Myrtaceae) significantly reduced formaline induced pain behaviour in mice and is often used is an analgesic and antiseptic in dental care. [19]

THYME ESSENTIAL OIL (THYMUS VULGARIS)

Investigation has shown that Thymus Vulgaris (TV) modulates pain.[20]

CUMIN KEY ESSENTIAL OIL(CUMINUM CYMINUM)

Findings suggest that cumin oil hold the potential to be applied for the treatment of inflammatory diseases. [21]

WILD ORANGE ESSENTIAL OIL

The Limonene content of Wild Orange essential oil has been found to have antidepressant like effects and would therefore be considered beneficial for use by people living with Fibromyalgia.[22]

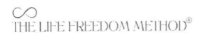
PEPPERMINT ESSENTIAL OIL(MENTA PIPERITA)

Peppermint oil is hugely versatile. The anti-inflammatory and antinociceptive effects of 3 types of Mentha were tested and the results showed statistically significant and dose-dependent anti-inflammatory and antinociceptive effects24

A study by published in 2019 25 demonstrated that topical irritants, such as and including peppermint oil may alleviate inflammatory muscle pain via activating cutaneous nociceptors and subsequently inhibiting the abnormal activity of muscular nociceptive neurons.

GINGER ROOT(ZINGIBER OFFICINALE) OIL

Ginger Root Oil has shown to have Antinociceptive effects in mice citing the possible reasons to be linked to induced antinociceptive activity was possibly related to its ability to inhibit glutamatergic system, TRPV1 receptors as well as through activation of l-arginine/nitric oxide/cGMP/protein kinase C/ATP-sensitive K+ channel pathway. [26]

CARAWAY SEED ESSENTIAL OIL

Combined treatment with peppermint and caraway oil modulates post- inflammatory visceral hyperalgesia synergistically.[27]

GERMAN CHAMOMILE ESSENTIAL OIL

Chamomile is commonly used due to its medicinal qualities contributed due to its make up of terpenoids and flavonoids. It is often used to support inflammation, muscle spasms and rheumatic pain.[28]

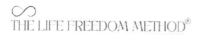
MICROPLEX VMZ

This supplement is a whole food formula of bioavailable vitamins and minerals that are deficient in our modern diet.[14]Many studies show that very few people meet the recommended dietary intakes for most vitamins and minerals. This supplement is a food nutrient complex which includes a balanced blend of essential antioxidant vitamins A, C and E, and an energy complex of B vitamins presented in a patented glycoprotein matrix (To make a vitamin glycoprotein compound, a vitamin is introduced to a culture of lactobacillus and yeast. As it grows, the yeast metabolises and binds the vitamin into its protein matrix, making the vitamin more recognisable as food in the digestive process.) They also include a full spectrum digestive enzyme blend of Peppermint, Ginger and carraway to support efficient digestion that also have other far reaching anti-inflammatory properties. [25 26 27 29]

This supplement provides 22 essential vitamins and minerals to support normal growth, function, and maintenance of cells:

- Fights free radicals with the antioxidant vitamins A, C, and E •Supports healthy metabolism and cellular energy
- Supports bone health with calcium, magnesium, zinc, and vitamin D •Supports healthy immune function
- Supports healthy digestion
- Provides systemic benefits of vitality and wellness associated with optimal intake of essential nutrients
- Methylated form of B9
- A balanced blend of essential vitamins including the antioxidant vitamins A, C, and E; an energy complex of B vitamins; presented in a patented glycoprotein matrix for enhanced bioavailability*
- Includes a balanced blend of chelated minerals including calcium, magnesium, zinc, selenium, copper, manganese, and chromium •Includes a whole-food botanical blend of kale, dandelion, parsley, kelp, broccoli, brussels, sprout, cabbage, and spinach
- Formulated with a digestive enzyme blend of protease, lactase, lipase, amylase, a-galactosidase, diastase, glucoamylase, and peptidase
- Contains a full-spectrum of vitamin E forms including tocotrienols

Vitamin D deficiency has been implicated in conditions like autoimmune and cardiovascular diseases, cancers, and chronic pain.[30]

It has also been found that there is a positive influence of B-vitamins on painful symptoms and indicate that less NSAID is needed for pain relief when combined with B-vitamins. [31]

ALPHA CRS+

Alpha CRS+ Cellular Vitality Complex is a proprietary formula combining potent levels of natural botanical extracts that support healthy cell function with important metabolic factors of cellular energy.

Alpha CRS + ® Cellular Vitality Complex is a proprietary dietary supplement formulated with potent levels of powerful polyphenols that support healthy cell function by providing antioxidant protection to cellular DNA and other critical cell structures. The cellular longevity polyphenol blend found in Alpha CRS+ includes concentrated extracts of baicalin from scutellaria root, which has been shown in studies to have anti-inflammatory effects.[32]

Resveratrol also an ingredient of this supplement has shown to have neurological recovery and anti-oxidant effects.[33]

Grape seeds have also been shown to have a positive impact on [34]
oxidative stress and inflammation. Curcumin from turmeric root [35] has been found to be an inflammation silencer. Silymarin from milk thistle supports the body's internal production of endogenous antioxidants such as glutathione. The blend also includes a proprietary blend of boswellic acid and bromelain protease enzyme that support healthy cellular function.

Coenzyme Q10, and a botanical extract of Ginko biloba to help support mental clarity and energy has also been found to have clinical improvement and a prominent reduction in pain fatigue, and morning tiredness. A reduction in the pain visual and a reduction in tender, including recovery of inflammation, antioxidant enzymes, mitochondrial biogenesis, and AMPK gene expression levels, associated with phosphorylation of the AMPK activity. These results lead to the hypothesis that CoQ have a potential therapeutic effect in Fibromyalgia and indicate new potential molecular targets for the therapy of this disease. AMPK could be implicated in the pathophysiology of Fibromyalgia.[36]

STEP 7

Patients were provided with a journal and asked to note down their thoughts and feelings as and when they felt like they wanted to. They were asked to make a note of any pain that they were experiencing and any positive changes in their quality of life. The benefits of journaling were explained to them based on experience and the findings of reports that show that written emotional expression produces health benefits. [32]

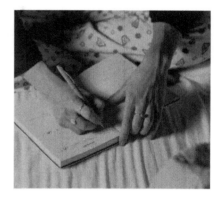

STEP 8

Meditation did not form a part of our subjects' regular daily activity before the pilot. Both pilot members were however provided with a 14-day educational meditation programme to follow and to then integrate this into their daily practice.

The reported cognitive and psychological benefits of meditation and mindfulness practice are well documented. Many of the benefits of mindfulness stem from the fact that the practice helps process thoughts without engaging with them.

It reduces stress and anxiety as patients become attuned to notice patterns of thinking or belief that give rise to stress or to observe a stressful feeling without ruminating.

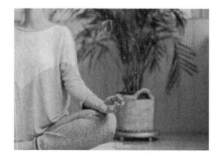

63

In 2013, researchers at the University of Montreal in Canada conducted review of more than 200 studies involving over 12,000 people and showed that mindfulness meditation is an effective treatment for a variety of psychological disorders, but that it was especially effective for reducing depression, anxiety and stress. All of which are required in the treatment of Fibromyalgia symptoms.[38]

Similarly, Johns Hopkins University researchers in the USA published a systematic review and meta-analysis in 2014 and 47 trials involving 3515 participants and concluded that meditation practice resulted in significant reduction in anxiety, depression and pain. They also suggested that include meditation practices as part of a wider treatment plan for optimising mental health.

Meditation can also be used in pain management. In 2020, a metaanalysis of 20 randomised controlled trials involving over 6000 participants published by researchers at the University of Utah showed that meditation and other Mind Body therapies for example, hypnosis, guided imagery and cognitive behavioural therapy, reduced acute pain, 40 chronic pain and post-surgical pain.

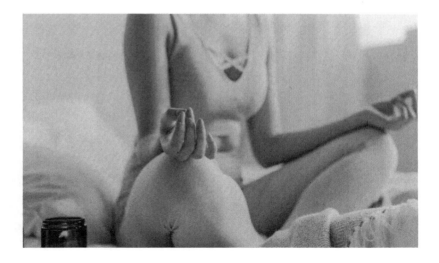

STEP 9

The demand for essential oils has been steadily growing over the years. This is mirrored by a substantial increase in research concerned with essential oils also in the field of inflammatory and neuropathic pain. A recent systematic review and meta-analysis investigated the preclinical evidence in favour of working hypothesis of the analgesic properties of essential oils elucidating whether there is a consistent rationale basis for translation into clinical setting. [68]

With education, the patients used different oils and oil blends for various psychological and physiological support at the outset of the 12-week programme which were bespoke to each of them and relating to the symptoms that they presented with at each consultation and before the trauma work at Step 10 commenced. Essential oils were used topically, internally and via inhalation. [13]

At the outset of the pilot both patients presented in a relatively stressed state. Hypertension was a diagnosed issue for one patient.

The results of a published review on The Effects of inhalation method [69] suggest that the inhalation method using essential oils can be considered an effective nursing intervention that reduces psychological stress responses and serum cortisol levels, as well as the blood pressure of clients with essential hypertension.

Aromatherapy was introduced as a way of preparing for rest. The bedtime routine involved the use of essential oils being diffused into the bedroom around 30 minutes before the patients went to bed. The oils used for sleep were Vetiver, Cedarwood and Lavender. The conditioned response that was being created signalled "time to relax".

Lavender has long been used to support sleep. A study by Smith et al,[70] found that the effect of inhaled lavender demonstrated better sleep quality postintervention. Lavender, cedarwood, and vetiver balms work as an anti-stress treatment by reducing plasma cortisol levels.

uyono, Jong and Wijaya[71] showed a reduction in plasma cortisol levels and can be used as an alternative medication to manage prolonged stress and aid sleep.
Other behavioural changes were introduced to patients in the current pilot, including phones off; no TV; no blue screens one hour before bed; magnesium salt baths with essential oils before bed.

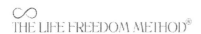
THE LIFE FREEDOM METHOD®

DEEP BLUE

Deep Blue" is an essential oil blend composed of Wintergreen, Camphor, Peppermint, Blue Tansy, German Chamomile, Helichrysum and Osmanthus oil. This was offered to support the reduction of inflammation directly on to the areas that were experiencing the sensations of pain. [72]

The study An essential oil blend significantly modulates immune responses and the cell cycle in human cell cultures; investigated The impact of essential oils on proteins associated with inflammation and tissue remodelling and on the genome-wide expression of 21,224 genes.

The study provided the first evidence indicating how these essential oils affect genome-wide gene expression in human skin cells and establishes a basis for further research into their biological mechanisms of action.
Deep Blue provided a potential alternative to the patients to pharmaceutical pain medicine.

FRANKINCENSE, MARJORAM, LEMON GRASS AND OREGANO

Frankincense, Marjoram, Lemongrass and Oregano in a veggie capsule and ingested with water.

There are a number of studies confirming the efficacy of this essential oil that comes from the resin of the Boswellia Serrata and the Boswellia carterii tree. The main component of frankincense is oil (60%). It contains mono (13%) and diterpenes (40%) as well as ethyl acetate (21.4%), octyl acetate (13.4%) and methylanisole (7.6%). The highest biological activity among terpenes is characteristic of 11-keto-ß-acetylbeta-boswellic acid, acetyl-11-keto-ß-boswellic acid and acetyl-α- boswellic acid.

Contemporary studies have shown that resin indeed have analgesic, tranquilising and anti-bacterial effects. From the point of view of therapeutic properties, extracts from Boswellia serrata and Boswellia carterii are reported to be particularly effective. They reduce inflammatory conditions in the course of rheumatism by inhibiting leukocyte elastase and degrading glycosaminoglycans.

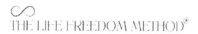

Boswellia preparations inhibit 5-lipoxygenase and prevent the release of leukotrienes, thus having an anti-inflammatory effect in ulcerative colitis, irritable bowel syndrome, bronchitis and sinusitis. Inhalation and consumption of Boswellia olibanum reduces the risk of asthma. In addition, boswellic acids have an antiproliferative effect on tumours. They inhibit proliferation of tumour cells of the leukaemia and glioblastoma subset. They have an anti-tumour effect since they inhibit topoisomerase I and II-alpha and stimulate programmed cell death (apoptosis).

Boswellic acids inhibited the production of pro-inflammatory IL-2 and IFN-γ (both Th1-related cytokines) but upregulated the production of anti-inflammatory/immunomodulatory IL-4 and IL-10 (both Th2-related cytokines) by murine splenic T cells.74 This Th1 to Th2 switch contributes to the anti-inflammatory and anti-arthritic effects of boswellic acids. In addition, AKBA has been shown to inhibit both Th17 differentiation and the production of cytokine IL-17 by these cells Two of the mechanisms relating to Th17 differentiation were identified as the targets in this process: inhibition of IL-1β signalling and STAT3 phosphorylation.

OREGANO ESSENTIAL OIL

There is evidence that mention that Oregano essential oil has the ability to exert anti-inflammatory activity. For example, Leyva-López et al [75] demonstrated that terpenes, such as thymol and carvacrol acetate, obtained from the three Mexican oregano species, L. graveolens, L. palmeri and H. patens reduced significantly the levels of ROS and NO produced by RAW 264.7 macrophage cells stimulated with lipopolysaccharide (LPS). Furthermore, EOs of O. majorana (10 µg/mL) reduced the production of tumor necrosis factor-alpha (TNF-α), interleukin-1β (IL-1β) and IL-6 in LPS-activated THP-1 human macrophage cells Recently, Han and Parker showed that EOs obtained from O. vulgare significantly inhibited the levels of the inflammatory biomarkers monocyte chemoattractan protein-1 (MCP-1), the vascular cell adhesion molecule-1 (VCAM-1) and the intracellular cell adhesion molecule-1 (ICAM-1) on activated-primary human neonatal fibroblasts. These findings suggest that the EOO have anti-inflammatory properties.

MARJORAM ESSENTIAL OIL

There are numerous studies supporting the use of essential oils and their ability to support the symptoms of pain. A study by the Korean Society of Nursing Sciences investigated Marjoram as well as several other oils.[76] Data clearly showed that aromatherapy had major effects on decreasing pain and depression levels. Based on the findings, it was suggested that aromatherapy can be a useful nursing intervention for arthritis patients.

LEMONGRASS ESSENTIAL OIL

Lemongrass Essential Oil was evaluated for its in vivo topical and oral anti-inflammatory effects. For the evaluation of the anti-inflammatory effect, LGEO (10 mg/kg, administered orally) significantly reduced carrageenan-induced paw oedema with a similar effect to that observed for oral diclofenac (50 mg/kg), which was used as the positive control. Oral administration of LGEO showed dose-dependent anti-inflammatory activity. [77]

COPAIBA ESSENTIAL OIL

This oil was given to be taken internally and topically when required. Copaiba has many useful properties for the body as well as impressive anti-inflammatory properties.[78] One study looked to evaluate the antihyperalgesic effect of the complex containing β-caryophyllene (βCP) and β-cyclodextrin (βCD) in a non-inflammatory chronic muscle pain mice model and investigated its action on superficial dorsal horn of the lumbar spinal cord. β-caryophyllene, a dietary cannabinoid, complexed with β- cyclodextrin produced anti-hyperalgesic effect involving the inhibition of Fos expression in superficial dorsal horn.

Key findings show the characterization tests indicated that βCP were efficiently incorporated into βCD. The oral treatment with βCP-βCD, at all doses tested, produced a significant ($p < 0.05$) reduction on mechanical hyperalgesia and a significant ($p < 0.05$) increase in muscle withdrawal thresholds, without produce any alteration in force. In addition, βCP-βCD was able to significantly ($p < 0.05$) decrease FOS expression in the superficial dorsal horn.[79] The biological activities of copaiba essential oil were determined to be fast acting, CB2 mediated, and dependent on multiple chemical constituents of the oil. Nanofluidic proteomics provided a powerful means to assess the biological activities of copaiba essential oil.

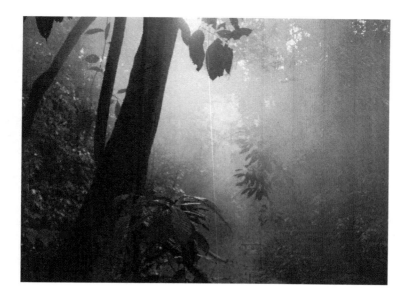

STEP 10

After 14 days from the initial introduction of steps 1-9, focus was shifted to the trauma response of the subjects.

Psychological and behavioural therapies are being applied to patients with fibromyalgia (FM) with increasing frequency. The rationale for including psychological therapies is not for the treatment of co-morbid mood disorders, but rather to manage the many non- psychiatric psychological and social factors that comprise pain perception and its maintenance.

Empirical literature supports the use of CBT with fibromyalgia in producing modest outcomes across multiple domains, including pain, fatigue, physical functioning and mood. Greatest benefits so far appear to occur when CBT is used adjunctively with exercise. While the benefits have not been curative or universally obtained by all patients, the benefits are sufficiently large to encourage future refinement of these combined therapies.

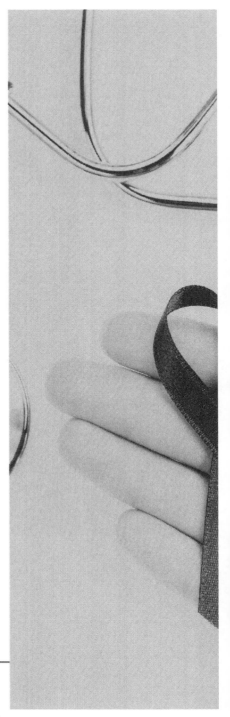

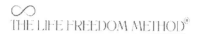
Most guidelines identify trauma-focused psychological treatments over pharmacological treatments as a preferred first step and view medications as an adjunct or a next line treatment. [41] Most options available to Fibromyalgia patients or those living with chronic pain are offered pharmaceutical opiate medication coupled with access to a pain management programme which teaches them to live and cope with the pain.

Belief Coding® is a method created by altruistic entrepreneur, Jessica Cunningham. The modality is fully accredited to help people work through and alter limiting beliefs and release trauma that is trapped inside the body.

Belief Coding® is made up of a number of scientifically validated modalities. It uses elements of Neuro Linguistic Programming (NLP); Hypnotherapy; Cognitive Behavioural Therapy, Emotional Freedom Technique (EFT), Meditation, Matrix Reimprinting, Kinesiology, energy healing, visualisation techniques and talking therapy. This can be supported with Reiki and Aromatherapy.

The Belief Coding® technique helps to remove the emotional charge from a past traumatic experience response, to allowing the patient to live free from pain by resolving the cellular memory of that trauma response experience.

It is widely recognised that a set of physiological and psychological processes become enacted when humans experience acute stress or [42] trauma. For many people, these physiological perturbations return to baseline once the stress or trauma has resolved. However, the initial state of hyperarousal can become chronic for some individuals. [43,44,45]

The chronic hyperarousal then leads to dysregulation of the physiologic stress system and the ultimate development of stress-related conditions. Consistent with cognitive behaviour theory, the experience of trauma also may impact one's appraisals of potentially threatening stimuli including physical and physiological symptoms. This appraisal bias may then lead to increased avoidance, catastrophizing about symptoms, and amplification of the illness experience [46] One's expectation of further somatic symptoms also can play a role in perpetuating a cycle of further decline in functioning. For example, an individual with Fibromyalgia may experience significant anticipatory anxiety associated with the likelihood of future pain which may cause him to isolate or limit his activity level, potentially leading to higher pain susceptibility and poorer psychosocial functioning. [47]

The Belief Coding® technique, in the main follows the following process.

APPLIED
KINESIOLOGY

In 1964 Dr George Goodheart Jr, introduced the concept of Applied Kinesiology. It is based on the idea that the body never lies. In the 1970's Dr John Diamond applied it to test the positive and negative effects of our thoughts have on the Thymus gland. It is a system used as a standard tool for practitioners who use muscle/energy testing to dialogue with the body. Muscle/energy testing is the response of our individual energy systems to the vibration of certain substances, people and statements/thoughts we make or have. Jessica Cunningham has used these principles and has adopted this as The Human Compass® to use at the start of the Belief Coding® technique process.

The purpose is to have the client/patient identify their body's yes and no response for us to begin to identify the trauma/discomfort that the body and the subconscious mind is ready to deal with. Once the discomfort has been identified from the list which has its base in The Emotion Code system.

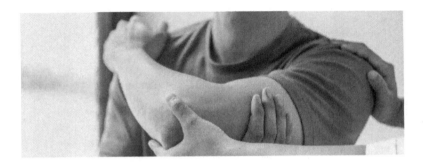

THE EMOTION CODE

The Emotion Code is an energy-based therapy that is used to identify, and release trapped emotional energy. It was developed by Dr Bradley Nelson over a 20-year period in his practice as a chiropractor. Jessica Cunningham has used the concept of the Emotions Chart used within Dr Nelson's Emotion Code practice and adapted it to encompass more emotions and discomforts as the Belief Coding® method has developed since its' inception in 2020. This coupled with the Human Compass® helps identify which discomfort/emotion will be worked on at any one time.

Once the emotion/discomfort is identified it is possible to pinpoint when the event/emotion happened and at what age the patient/client was at that time by using the Human Compass®.
Emotional Freedom Technique (EFT)

Meta- Analysis suggests that Clinical EFT improves multiple physiological markers of health. In particular, the considerable reduction of the experience of pain has been noted within two studies for Chronic Illness and Fibromyalgia. Emotional freedom techniques (EFT) as a practice for supporting chronic disease healthcare: a practitioners' perspective [49] and Self-administered EFT (Emotional Freedom Techniques) in individuals with fibromyalgia.[50]

By tapping on the acupuncture meridian points, coupled with the Human Compass identifying the emotion/discomfort and age helps the subconscious mind bring forward a reflection/memory that the emotion/discomfort is linked to.

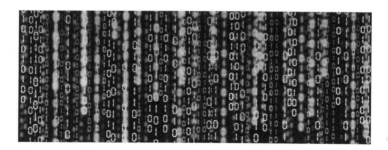

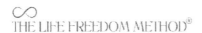
THE LIFE FREEDOM METHOD®

REFLECTION: AUTOBIOGRAPHICAL MEMORY (A M) & EPISODIC MEMORY

Autobiographical memory is a complex blend of memories of single, recurring, and extended events integrated into a coherent story of self that is created and evaluated through sociocultural practices. It entails a complex set of operations, including episodic memory, self-reflection, emotion, visual imagery, attention, executive functions, and semantic processes.

Episodic memory refers to a neurocognitive system that renders possible the conscious recollection of events as they were previously experienced. A key study 51 provides insight into the various parts of the brain responsible for the process of memory recall and how it can be harnessed to alter personal perspectives.

When looking at the function of working memory (WM) and autobiographical memory (AM) in patients with chronic pain, patients with chronic pain score significantly lower in the working memory index and higher in the Autobiographical Memory Test (AMT).[52]

Therefore, a working hypothesis is that by working with the Autobiographical Memory (Including the episodic Memory), we are able to alter the perception of that pain and bring that new reality in to the Working Memory Index. It is possible therefore this is further reflected in blood antibodies.

Since Freud, clinicians have understood that disturbing memories contribute to psychopathology and that new emotional experiences contribute to therapeutic change. Yet, controversy remains about what is truly essential to bring about psychotherapeutic change. Mounting evidence from empirical studies suggests that emotional arousal is a key ingredient in therapeutic change in many modalities. In addition, memory seems to play an important role but there is a lack of consensus on the role of understanding what happened in the past in bringing about therapeutic change.

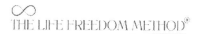

The core rationale in Belief Coding® is that therapeutic change in a variety of modalities, including behavioural therapy, cognitive- behavioural therapy, emotion-focused therapy, Neuro linguistic programming, talking therapy and psychodynamic psychotherapy, results from the updating of prior emotional memories through a process of reconsolidation that incorporates new emotional experiences.

This model uses 3 main elements:

Autobiographical (event) memories, semantic structures, and emotional responses supported by emerging evidence from cognitive neuroscience on implicit and explicit emotion, implicit and explicit memory, emotion memory interactions, memory reconsolidation, and the relationship between autobiographical and semantic memory. Belief Coding® identifies the vital parts of the process required for therapeutic change to take place. Firstly, reactivating old memories in a Trauma Informed environment.

Secondly incorporating new emotional experiences within this reactivated memory via the process of reconsolidation. Where necessary, using visualization techniques to alter the perception of physical pain within that memory. [53]The reconsolidation process includes the use of visualisation techniques.

It is now well understood that visualisation techniques is an optimum way of enhancing performance in any sport or movement by combining movement with the specific visualisation and neuroscience has shown that visualization has helped many people recover from stroke faster than standard interventions. ^Further analysis suggests that visualisation even helps to repair some damaged pain regions, and in some others the area responsible for movement switches to an undamaged area of the brain, permitting neuroplasticity and a return to more able movement.

The immune system has also been found to respond to visualisation. Researchers at the UK Lincolnshire Hospital NHS Trust in the UK conducted a randomized controlled trial for women receiving treatment for breast cancer. Each woman within the randomized visualisation group visualized her immune system destroying the cancel cells.

They used whichever visualisation that worked for them. From piranha fish to Pac-man. The women who visualized this destruction were found to have much higher levels of key immune cells, killer (NK) cells, T cells and T helper cells than those that did not visualize. This was after four rounds of chemotherapy.

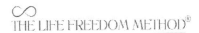

THE LIFE FREEDOM METHOD®

The published with The Breast journal, researchers reported that the immune system was still showing high cytotoxicity against cancer cells after the four cycles, but only in the women who were visualizing their immune cells destroying the cancer cells.[56, 57]

Thirdly, reinforcing the new integrated memory structure by way of matrix reimprinting, an energy psychology using quantum physics, by practicing a new way of behaving and experiencing life.

Within the Belief Coding® process we use the modality of guided visualisation to remove the pain from the body in a similar way to the piranha and Pac-Man analogy. The Belief Coding® technique allows the patient to work with each trauma as it comes up for them. This helps us break down the complex narratives in a way that allows the patient to work through each aspect at their own pace.

Pascua I-Leone & Greenberg[58] proposes a sequential order of shifting from "early expressions of distress" to "primary adaptive emotion" that aid in adaptive functioning. The model of emotional processing study tested a model of emotional processes over the course of emotion-focused therapy for trauma. Thirty-eight participants were taken from a randomized clinical trial to examine in-session process from video recordings of treatment. The sample had an average age (M = 44.3 years) and the majority was female (55.3%) and of European descent (89.5%). The Classification of Affective Meaning States was used to examine changes in emotional processes during trauma narratives in both early and late sessions. Findings have implications for guiding therapeutic process in a productive manner that leads to trauma recovery. Changes in discrete emotions were related to good treatment outcome.

It is also more effective to work with each patient in an individual capacity rather than in a group environment. The nature of the openness of the communication between patient and facilitator does not lend itself to a group environment. Whilst this is particularly valid in this scenario, Meta-Ana lysis of psychological treatments for PTSD in adult survivors of childhood abuse, shows that individua trauma focused therapy has better outcomes.[59]

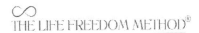

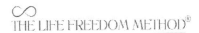

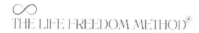

Furthermore, whilst working in a trauma informed way, studies have also examined observable moment by moment steps in emotional processing as they occurred within productive sessions of experiential therapy.[60] These investigation consisted of 2 studies as part of a task analysis that examined clients processing distress in live video-recorded therapy sessions. Clients in both studies were adults in experiential therapy for depression and ongoing interpersonal problems. Study 1 was the discovery-oriented phase of task analysis, which intensively examined 6 examples of global distress. The qualitative findings produced a model showing: global distress, fear, shame, and aggressive anger as undifferentiated and insufficiently processed emotions; the articulation of needs and negative self-evaluations as a pivotal step in change; and assertive anger, self-soothing, hurt, and grief as states of advanced processing. Study 2 tested the model using a sample of 34 clients in global distress. A multivariate analysis of variance showed that the model of emotional processing predicted positive in-session effects, and bootstrapping analyses were used to demonstrate that distinct emotions emerged moment by moment in predicted sequential patterns. This is the way in which we break down each traumatic response relating to metaphysical pain and beliefs in the Belief Coding® technique.

REIKI

Reiki, whilst not too long ago was considered completely woo, Reiki is now becoming accepted as a viable practice within some UK hospitals and private practice (The Christie, Manchester, by way of example)

There are growing numbers of scientific studies that show it can be effective. Studies have demonstrated that reiki can help to reduce pain, anxiety, depression and blood pressure in patients that have experienced various interventions, including cancer, knee replacements, hysterectomy, back pain for example.

A 2018 meta analysis[61]of four randomized controlled studies into the use of using Reiki for reducing pains across a number of conditions showed that it supported a significant reduction in pain. A further paper [62] published in the BMJ Supportive & Palliative Care 2019 concluded that reiki therapy is useful for relieving pain, decreasing anxiety and depression and improving quality of life in certain conditions.

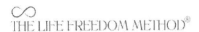

By way of using Reiki as a complimentary therapy, Reiki and physiotherapy were compared with drug treatment for relieving lower back pain. Both Reiki and Physiotherapy significantly reduced levels of pain and were much more effective than drug treatment.

POSITIVE AFFIRMATIONS

The visualisation process at the end of the "pain removal" element of the Belief Coding® process is cemented by the reimprinting of a new belief by way of repetition of a positive affirmation chosen by the patient.

This repetition coupled with the visualisation of life without the particular area of pain or with the self-limiting belief has been shown to influence the brain networks, shaping them in the direction of producing what the brain is visualizing. The Psychology Dictionary defines an affirmation as "a brief phrase which is spoken again and again in an effort to plant seeds of happy and positive notions, conceptions and attitudes into one's psyche"

Claude Steele, published a paper[64] on his self-affirmation theory. The premise of which states that humans are fundamentally motivated to maintain a positive self-view. A general perception of ourselves that we are good, stable, capable people with a freedom of choice and a sense of control over important outcomes in our lives.

These self-affirmations then affirm our core values. By doing this research shows that this creates the ability to adopt a more positive mindset and are much more likely to indulge in healthy behaviours and taking positive steps to improve life. This is especially the case when these affirmations are repeated regularly.

This is a vital part of the whole process. It helps with consistency of life after the "treatment" and helps with the nutrition element of the Life Freedom Method®. A study at the University of Sheffield.[65] found that changes in healthy behaviour also applied to diet. This is key for everyone but absolutely for people living with Fibromyalgia. Education + Affirmations is a positive integral part of the care plan.

PRELIMINARY RESULTS

Data indicates that health profiles for both pilot participants made significant positive shifts across all three measurement points (Fig 1).

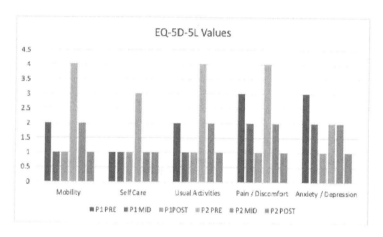

Fig 1 – EQ5D5L Profile changes across three time points.

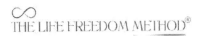
Positive changes were also achieved in the self-rated health index which scores from 0 - 100 representing poor health and good health respectively (Fig 2).

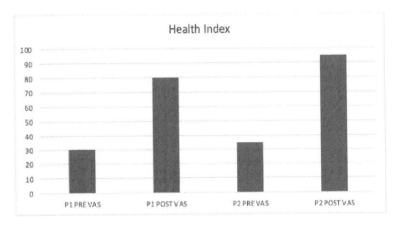

Fig 2 – VAS self-rating for perception of health today.

When data from EQ5D5L was transformed into utility values it demonstrated an improvement of 25% and 70% for participants 1 and 2 respectively (Fig 3). Changes in QALY over time can be viewed in Fig 4.

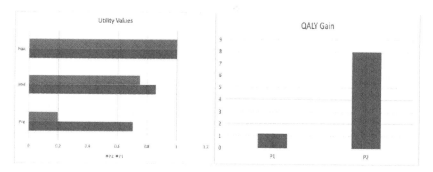

Fig 3 – Utility values and QALY changes pre and post for participants 1 and 2.

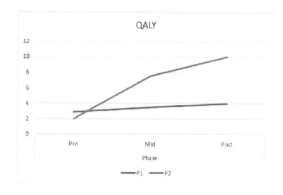

Fig 4 – Individual QALY changes over three time points

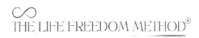

The pilot study also evaluated changes in the brain pain inventory over three time points. Table 1 indicates positive improvement consistently over time.

Table 1 - Changes in brain pain inventory over three time points.

		Brain Pain Inventory					
		P1			P2		
	Questions	Week 1	Mid Term	Week 12	Week 1	Mid Term	Week 12
Q1	Have you had pain other than everyday kinds of pain today	YES	YES	NO	YES	YES	YES
Q2	On the diagram shade in areas where you feel pain	Whole Body		Shoulders/arms/wrist	Whole Body	Sternum	Right Knee
Q3	Please rate pain at its worst today	8	3	1	9	3	4
Q4	Please rate pain at its least today	5	2	1	8	0	0
Q5	Please rate average pain today	6	2	1	7	2	2
Q6	Please rate pain right now	7	2	1	7	0	2
Q7	What treatments or medications are you receiving for your pain	Pregabalin 600mg, Sertraline, Paracetamol	Pregabalin 300mg, sertraline	Pregabalin 150mg Sertraline	Codeine Paracetemol, Naproxen, Sertraline, Lesatin, Omeprazole	Sertraline. Lesatin, Omeprazole	Sertraline, lesatin
Q8	How much relief have you had from your pain medication	10%	10%	0%	90%	0%	0%
Q9	How has pain interfered in the last 24 hours with General activity	7	0	0	8	2	0
	How has pain interfered in the last 24 hours with Mood	8	4	0	7	2	0
	How has pain interfered in the last 24 hours with walking ability	7	0	0	7	3	4
	How has pain interfered in the last 24 hours with normal work	3	1	0	7	3	0
	How has pain interfered in the last 24 hours with relations with others	2	2	0	8	2	0
	How has pain interfered in the last 24 hours with sleep	7	1	0	8	5	0
	How has pain interfered in the last 24 hours with enjoyment of life	6	1	0	8	1	0

CONCLUSION

The pilot trial of The Life Freedom Method® has generated evidence to support the reduction of pain and improvement in quality of life. To date it is yet to be demonstrated that there is a link between The Life Freedom Method® treatment approach has impacted the specific binding of antibodies to the cells within the Dorsal Root Ganglia.

This document indicates that there is strong evidence supporting the individual components that comprise the Life Freedom Method®

Whilst the evidence is compelling for each of the programme elements, no work exists that evaluates them in combination as a single treatment option for chronic pain management in Fibromyalgia.

Preliminary results from a pilot investigation provide promising insight into the effectiveness of the programme and further work is warranted on a larger scale to determine if the results are replicable across a larger controlled cohort.

For more information please contact Jules Kelly - Space and Freedom Limited 07368 256717

REFERENCES

1. https://www.jci.org/articles/view/144201/

2. Thomas, K.B. (1987) "General practice consultations: is there any point in being positive?" British Medical Journal, 294 (6581),pp1200-1202

3. Frans Derksen, Jozien Bensing and Antoine Lagro-Janssen British Journal of General Practice 2013; 63 (606): e76-e84.

4. De la Fuente-Fernández, R.,et al (2017) "Expectation and dopamine release: mechanism of the placebo effect in Parkinsons' disease', Science, 293 (5532), pp. 1164-1166

5. Benedetti, F., et al (2016) "Teaching neurons to respond to placebos". Journal of Physiology, 594 (19), pp5647-5660

6. Chen, X., Zou, K., Abdullah, N. et al. The placebo effect and its determinants in fibromyalgia: meta-analysis of randomised controlled trials. Clin Rheumatol 36, 1623–1630 (2017). https://doi.org/10.1007/s10067-017-3595-8

7. Robert John Adams (2010) Improving health outcomes with better patient understanding and education, Risk Management and Healthcare Policy, 3:, 61-72, DOI: 10.2147/RMHP.S7500

8 MurrayEBurnsJSee TaiSLaiRNazarethIInteractive health communication applications for people with chronic diseaseCochrane Database Syst Rev20054CD00427416235356

9. PortnoyDBScott-SheldonLAJJohnsonBTCareyMPComputer-delivered interventions for health promotion and behavioral risk reduction: a meta-analysis of 75 randomized controlled trials, 1988–2007Prev Med20084731618403003

10. Rowena Field, M. Physio, Fereshteh Pourkazemi, PhD, Jessica Turton, Kieron Rooney, PhD, Dietary Interventions Are Beneficial for Patients with Chronic Pain: A Systematic Review with Meta-Analysis, Pain Medicine, Volume 22, Issue 3, March 2021, Pages 694–714, https://doi.org/10.1093/pm/pnaa378

11   Rodriguez B, Hochstrasser A, Eugster PJ, Grouzmann E, Müri RM, Z'Graggen WJ. Brain fog in neuropathic postural tachycardia syndrome may be associated with autonomic hyperarousal and improves after water drinking. Front Neurosci. 2022 Aug 5;16:968725. doi: 10.3389/fnins.2022.968725. PMID: 35992935; PMCID: PMC9388780.

12 Elma Ö, Yilmaz ST, Deliens T, Coppieters I, Clarys P, Nijs J, et al. Do nutritional factors interact with chronic musculoskeletal pain? A systematic review. J Clin Med. 2020;9(3):702.

13 Haddad, H.W., Mallepalli, N.R., Scheinuk, J.E. et al. The Role of Nutrient Supplementation in the Management of Chronic Pain in Fibromyalgia: A Narrative Review. Pain Ther 10, 827–848 (2021). https://doi.org/10.1007/s40122- 021-00266-9

14 Loren Cordain, S Boyd Eaton, Anthony Sebastian, Neil Mann, Staffan Lindeberg, Bruce A Watkins, James H O'Keefe, Janette Brand-Miller, Origins and evolution of the Western diet: health implications for the 21st century, The American Journal of Clinical Nutrition, Volume 81, Issue 2, February 2005, Pages 341–354, https://doi.org/10.1093/ajcn.81.2.341

15 Calder PC. Marine omega-3 fatty acids and inflammatory processes: Effects, mechanisms and clinical relevance. Biochim Biophys Acta. 2015 Apr;1851(4):469-84. doi: 10.1016/j.bbalip.2014.08.010. Epub 2014 Aug 20. PMID: 25149823.

16 Selected CAM Therapies for Arthritis-Related Pain: The Evidence From Systematic Reviews Soeken, Karen L. PhD The Clinical Journal of Pain 20(1):p 13-18, January 2004.

17 Calder, P. (2013). N-3 Fatty acids, inflammation and immunity: New mechanisms to explain old actions. Proceedings of the Nutrition Society, 72(3), 326-336. doi:10.1017/S0029665113001031

18 Lombardo, Mauro, Alessandra Feraco, Morena Ottaviani, Gianluca Rizzo, Elisabetta Camajani, Massimiliano Caprio, and Andrea Armani. 2022. "The Efficacy of Vitamin D Supplementation in the Treatment of Fibromyalgia Syndrome and Chronic Musculoskeletal Pain" Nutrients 14, no. 15: 3010. https://doi.org/10.3390/nu14153010

19 (Halder et al 2012 Halder S, Mehta AK, Mediratta PK, Sharma KK. Acute effect of essential oil of Eugenia caryophyllata on cognition and pain in mice. Naunyn Schmiedebergs Arch Pharmacol. 2012 Jun;385(6):587-93. doi: 10.1007/s00210-012-0742-2. Epub 2012 Mar 28. PMID: 22453493.

20 Abbas Ali Taherian et al.; antinociceptive effects of hydroalcoholic extract of Thymus vulgaris. Pak. J. Pharm. Sci., Vol.22, No.1, January 2009, pp.83-89.

21 https://www.frontiersin.org/articles/10.3389/fphar.2021.674095/full
ORIGINAL RESEARCH article
Front. Pharmacol., 11 October 2021 Sec.
Ethnopharmacology
Volume 12 - 2021 | https://doi.org/10.3389/fphar.2021.674095

22 Antidepressant-like Effect of Citrus sinensis (L.) Osbeck Essential Oil and Its Main Component Limonene on Mice Lu-Lu Zhang, Zi-Yu Yang, Gang Fan, Jing-Nan Ren, Kai-Jing Yin, and Si-Yi PanJournal of Agricultural and Food Chemistry 2019 67 (50), 13817-13828

23 Susanna Stea, Alina Beraudi, Dalila De Pasquale, "Essential Oils for Complementary Treatment of Surgical Patients: State of the Art", Evidence-Based Complementary and Alternative Medicine, vol. 2014, Article ID 726341, 6 pages, 2014. https://doi.org/10.1155/2014/726341

24 Mogosan C, Vostinaru O, Oprean R, Heghes C, Filip L, Balica G, Moldovan RI. A Comparative Analysis of the Chemical Composition, Anti-Inflammatory, and Antinociceptive Effects of the Essential Oils from Three Species of Mentha Cultivated in Romania. Molecules. 2017; 22(2):263. https://doi.org/10.3390/molecules22020263

24 Mogosan C, Vostinaru O, Oprean R, Heghes C, Filip L, Balica G, Moldovan RI. A Comparative Analysis of the Chemical Composition, Anti-Inflammatory, and Antinociceptive Effects of the Essential Oils from Three Species of Mentha Cultivated in Romania. Molecules. 2017; 22(2):263. https://doi.org/10.3390/molecules22020263

25 Fang, Y., Zhu, J., Duan, W. et al. Inhibition of Muscular Nociceptive Afferents via the Activation of Cutaneous Nociceptors in a Rat Model of Inflammatory Muscle Pain. Neurosci. Bull. 36, 1–10 (2020). https://doi.org/10.1007/s12264-019-00406-4

26 Mohamed Hanief Khalid, Muhammad Nadeem Akhtar, Azam Shah Mohamad, Enoch Kumar Perimal, Ahmad Akira, Daud Ahmad Israf, Nordin Lajis, Mohd Roslan Sulaiman,
Antinociceptive effect of the essential oil of Zingiber zerumbet in mice: Possible mechanisms, Journal of Ethnopharmacology,
Volume 137, Issue 1,
2011,
Pages 345-351,
ISSN 0378-8741,
https://doi.org/10.1016/j.jep.2011.05.043.

27 Adam B, Liebregts T, Best J, Bechmann L, Lackner C, Neumann J, Koehler S, Holtmann G. A combination of peppermint oil and caraway oil attenuates the post-inflammatory visceral hyperalgesia in a rat model. Scand J Gastroenterol. 2006 Feb;41(2):155-60. doi: 10.1080/00365520500206442. PMID: 16484120.

28 Chicago Srivastava, J. K., Shankar, E., Gupta, S."Chamomile: A herbal medicine of the past with a bright future (Review)". Molecular Medicine Reports 3, no. 6 (2010): 895-901. https://doi.org/10.3892/mmr.2010.377

29 Gomez-Pinilla F, Gomez AG. The influence of dietary factors in central nervous system plasticity and injury recovery. PM R. 2011 Jun;3(6 Suppl 1):S111-6. doi: 10.1016/j.pmrj.2011.03.001. PMID: 21703566; PMCID: PMC3258094.

30 Sebastian Straube, R. Andrew Moore, Sheena Derry, Henry J. McQuay,
Vitamin D and chronic pain,
PAIN®, Volume 141, Issues 1–2, 2009, Pages 10-13, ISSN 0304-3959, https://doi.org/10.1016/j.pain.2008.11.010. (https://www.sciencedirect.com/science/article/pii/S0304395908007069)

31 Vetter G, Brüggemann G, Lettko M, et al. [Shortening diclofenac therapy by B vitamins. Results of a randomized double-blind study, diclofenac 50 mg versus diclofenac 50 mg plus B vitamins, in painful spinal diseases with degenerative changes]. Zeitschrift fur Rheumatologie. 1988 Sep-Oct;47(5):351-362. PMID: 3071032.

32 (Rosenbaum, Cathy Creger, Dónal P. O'Mathána, Mary Chavez, and Kelly Shields. "Antioxidants and antiinflammatory dietary supplements for osteoarthritis and rheumatoid arthritis." Alternative Therapies in Health & Medicine 16, no. 2 (2010).

33 (Xu BP, Yao M, Li ZJ, Tian ZR, Ye J, Wang YJ, Cui XJ. Neurological recovery and antioxidant effects of resveratrol in rats with spinal cord injury: a meta-analysis. Neural Regen Res. 2020 Mar;15(3):482-490. doi: 10.4103/1673-5374.266064. PMID: 31571660; PMCID: PMC6921347.)

34 (The effect of grape seed extract supplementation on oxidative stress and inflammation: A systematic review and meta-analysis of controlled trials
Sahar Foshati, Mohammad Hossein Rouhani, Reza AmaniFirst published: 09 June 2021
https://doi.org/10.1111/ijcp.14469,

35(Shima Hasanzadeh, Morgayn I. Read, Abigail R. Bland, Muhammed Majeed, Tannaz Jamialahmadi, Amirhossein Sahebkar,Curcumin: an inflammasome silencer, Pharmacological Research,Volume 159,202 104921

36 Can Coenzyme Q10 Improve Clinical and Molecular Parameters in Fibromyalgia?
Mario D. Cordero, Elísabet Alcocer-Gómez, Manuel de Miguel, Ognjen Culic, Angel M. Carrión, José Miguel Alvarez- Suarez, Pedro Bullón, Maurizio Battino, Ana Fernández-Rodríguez, and José Antonio Sánchez-Alcazar
Antioxidants & Redox Signaling 2013 19:12, 1356-1361

37 Broderick, Joan E. PhD; Junghaenel, Doerte U. MA; Schwartz, Joseph E. PhD. Written Emotional Expression Produces Health Benefits in Fibromyalgia Patients. Psychosomatic Medicine 67(2):p 326-334, March 2005. | DOI: 10.1097/01.psy.0000156933.04566.bd

38 Bassam Khoury, Tania Lecomte, Guillaume Fortin, Marjolaine Masse, Phillip Therien, Vanessa Bouchard, Marie-Andrée Chapleau, Karine Paquin, Stefan G. Hofmann,
Mindfulness-based therapy: A comprehensive meta-analysis, Clinical
Psychology Review, Volume 33, Issue 6, 2013, Pages 763-771,
ISSN 0272-7358, https://doi.org/10.1016/j.cpr.2013.05.005.

39. Goyal, M., Singh, S., Sibinga, E.M., Gould, N.F., Rowland-Seymour, A., Sharma, R., Berger, Z., Sleicher, D., Maron, D.D., Shihab, H.M. and Ranasinghe, P.D., 2014. Meditation programs for psychological stress and well-being: a systematic review and meta-analysis. JAMA internal medicine, 174(3), pp.357-368.

40 Garland EL, Brintz CE, Hanley AW, et al. Mind-Body Therapies for Opioid-Treated Pain: A Systematic Review and Meta-analysis. JAMA Intern Med. 2020;180(1):91–105. doi:10.1001/jamainternmed.2019.4917

41(American Psychiatric Association, 2004; Australian National Health and Medical Research Council (NHMRC) Guidelines, & Australian Centre for Posttraumatic Mental Health, 2007; National Institute for Health and Clinical Excellence, 2005, VA/DoD Clinical Practice Guideline Working Group, 2004.

42 Delvaux M, Denis P, Allemand H. Sexual abuse is more frequently reported by IBS patients than by patients with organic digestive diseases or controls. Results of a multicentre inquiry. French Club of Digestive Motility. Eur J Gastroenterol Hepatol. 1997;9:345–52

43 Ciccone DS, Elliott DK, Chandler HK, Nayak S, Raphael KG. Sexual and Physical Abuse in Women With Fibromyalgia Syndrome: A Test of the Trauma Hypothesis. The Clinical Journal of Pain. 2005;21:378–86.

44Clark C, Goodwin L, Stansfeld SA, Hotopf M, White PD. Premorbid risk markers for chronic fatigue syndrome in the 1958 British birth cohort. Br J Psychiatry. 2011;199:323–9.

45Koloski NA, Talley NJ, Boyce PM. A history of abuse in community subjects with irritable bowel syndrome and functional dyspepsia: the role of other psychosocial variables. Digestion. 2005;72:86–96.

46 Liebschutz J, Saitz R, Brower V, Keane TM, Lloyd-Travaglini C, Averbuch T, Samet JH. PTSD in urban primary care: high prevalence and low physician recognition. J Gen Intern Med. 2007;22:719–26

47 Afari N, Ahumada SM, Wright LJ, Mostoufi S, Golnari G, Reis V, Cuneo JG. Psychological trauma and functional somatic syndromes: a systematic review and meta-analysis. Psychosom Med. 2014 Jan;76(1):2-11. doi: 10.1097/PSY.0000000000000010. Epub 2013 Dec 12. PMID: 24336429; PMCID: PMC3894419.

48 Bach, D., Groesbeck, G., Stapleton, P., Sims, R., Blickheuser, K. and Church, D., 2019. Clinical EFT (Emotional Freedom Techniques) improves multiple physiological markers of health. Journal of evidence-based integrative medicine, 24, p.2515690X18823691.

49 Kalla M, Simmons M, Robinson A, Stapleton P. Emotional freedom techniques (EFT) as a practice for supporting chronic disease healthcare: a practitioners' perspective. Disabil Rehabil. 2018;40: 1654-1662. doi:10.1080/09638288.2017.1306125 34.

50 Brattberg G. Self-administered EFT (Emotional Freedom Techniques) in individuals with fibromyalgia in a randomized trial. Integr Med. 2008;7:30-35. 35

51 Eva Svoboda, Margaret C. McKinnon, Brian Levine,
The functional neuroanatomy of autobiographical memory: A meta-analysis, Neuropsychologia, Volume 44, Issue 12, 2006, Pages 2189-2208, ISSN 0028-3932,
https://doi.org/10.1016/j.neuropsychologia.2006.05.023.

52 Xianhua Liu, Hong Yang, Sisi Li, Di Wan, Yu Deng, Yonghui Fu, Qiong Qu, Linying Zhong & Yiqiu Hu (2021) Mediating effects of working memory on the relationship between chronic pain and overgeneral autobiographical memory, Memory, 29:3, 298-304, DOI: 10.1080/09658211.2021.1889606

53 M. Piñeyro, R.I. Ferrer Monti, H. Díaz, A.M. Bueno, S.G. Bustos, V.A. Molina, Positive emotional induction interferes with the reconsolidation of negative autobiographical memories, in women only, Neurobiology of Learning and Memory, Volume 155, 2018, Pages 508-518, ISSN 1074-7427,

54 Vinoth K. Ranganathan, Vlodek Siemionow, Jing Z. Liu, Vinod Sahgal, Guang H. Yue,From mental power to muscle power—gaining strength by using the mind, Neuropsychologia,Volume 42, Issue 7,2004,Pages 944-956, ISSN 0028-3932,https://doi.org/10.1016/j.neuropsychologia.2003.11.018.

55 Andrew J. Butler, Stephen J. Page, Mental Practice With Motor Imagery: Evidence for Motor Recovery and Cortical Reorganization After Stroke, Archives of Physical Medicine and Rehabilitation, Volume 87, Issue 12, Supplement, 2006,Pages 2-11,ISSN 0003-9993, https://doi.org/10.1016/j.apmr.2006.08.326.

56 Oleg Eremin, Mary B. Walker, Edna Simpson, Steven D. Heys, Antoine K. Ah-See, Andrew W. Hutcheon, Keith N. Ogston, Tarun K. Sarkar, Ashok Segar, Leslie G. Walker,

57 The Breast, Volume 18, Issue 1, 2009, Pages 17-25, ISSN 0960-9776, https://doi.org/10.1016/j.breast.2008.09.002.

58 Khayyat-Abuaita, U., Paivio, S., Pascual-Leone, A., & Harrington, S. (2019). Emotional processing of trauma narratives is a predictor of outcome in emotion-focused therapy for complex trauma. Psychotherapy, 56(4), 526–536. https://doi.org/10.1037/pst0000238

59 Individual Trauma Focused Therapy has a better outcome on PTSD
Thomas Ehring, Renate Welboren, Nexhmedin Morina, Jelte M. Wicherts, Janina Freitag, Paul M.G. Emmelkamp,Meta-analysis of psychological treatments for posttraumatic stress disorder in adult survivors of childhood abuse, Clinical Psychology Review, Volume 34, Issue 8, 2014, Pages 645-657, ISSN 0272-7358, https://doi.org/10.1016/j.cpr.2014.10.004.

60 Pascual-Leone A, Greenberg LS. Emotional processing in experiential therapy: why "the only way out is through.". J Consult Clin Psychol. 2007 Dec;75(6):875-87. doi: 10.1037/0022-006X.75.6.875. PMID: 18085905.

61 Melike Demir Doğan,
The effect of reiki on pain: A meta-analysis, Complementary Therapies in Clinical Practice, Volume 31, 2018, Pages 384-387,ISSN 1744-3881, https://doi.org/10.1016/j.ctcp.2018.02.020

62 Billot M, Daycard M, Wood C, et al
Reiki therapy for pain, anxiety and quality of life BMJ Supportive & Palliative Care 2019;9:434-438.

63 Jahantiqh, F., Abdollahimohammad, A., Firouzkouhi, M. and Ebrahiminejad, V., 2018. Effects of Reiki versus physiotherapy on relieving lower back pain and improving activities daily living of patients with intervertebral disc hernia. Journal of evidence-based integrative medicine, 23, p.2515690X18762745.

64 Claude M. Steele,
The Psychology of Self-Affirmation: Sustaining the Integrity of the Self, Editor(s): Leonard Berkowitz, Advances in Experimental Social Psychology, Academic Press, Volume 21,1988, Pages 261-302, ISSN 0065-2601,

65 Epton, T., & Harris, P. R. (2008). Self-affirmation promotes health behavior change. Health Psychology, 27(6), 746–752. https://doi.org/10.1037/0278-6133.27.6.746

66 Kim ES, Chen Y, Nakamura JS, Ryff CD, VanderWeele TJ. Sense of Purpose in Life and Subsequent Physical, Behavioral, and Psychosocial Health: An Outcome-Wide Approach. American Journal of Health Promotion. 2022;36(1):137-147. doi:10.1177/08901171211038545

67. Cummins, Robert & Woerner, Jacqueline & Gibson, Adele & Lai, Lufanna & Weinberg, Melissa & Collard, James. (2008). Australian Unity Wellbeing Index: Survey 20.

68 Efficacy of Essential Oils in Pain: A Systematic Review and Meta-Analysis of Preclinical Evidence Sec. Inflammation Pharmacology
Volume 12 - 2021 | https://doi.org/10.3389/fphar.2021.640128

69 The Effects of the Inhalation Method Using Essential Oils on Blood Pressure and Stress Responses of Clients with Essential Hypertension Journal of Korean Academy of Nursing 2006; 36(7): 1123-1134. Published online: 31 December 2006 DOI: https://doi.org/10.4040/jkan.2006.36.7.1123

70 Angela Smith Lillehei, etx al. A Randomized controlled trial . the Journal of Alternative and Complimentary Medicine July 2015 430-438

71 Rajasekhar CH, Kokila BN, Rajesh B. Potential effect of Vetiveria zizanoides root extract and essential oil on phenobarbital induced sedation-hypnosis in swiss albino mice, Int J Exp Pharmacol. 2014; 4:89-93

72 Han X, Parker TL. Essential oils diversely modulate genome-wide gene expression in human dermal fibroblasts. Cogent Medicine (2017)4(1). https://www.tandfonline.com/doi/full/10.1080/2331205X.2017.1307591

73 Boswellic acids is the active principle in treatment of chronic inflammatory diseases Wien Med Wochenschr 2002;152(15-16):373-8 doi: 10.1046/j.1563-258x.2002.02056.x. https://www.sciencedirect.com/science/article/abs/pii/S1744388122000962

74 Moudgil KD, Venkatesha SH. The Anti-Inflammatory and Immunomodulatory Activities of Natural Products to Control Autoimmune Inflammation. International Journal of Molecular Sciences. 2023; 24(1):95. https://doi.org/10.3390/ijms24010095

75 Leyva-López N, Gutiérrez-Grijalva EP, Vazquez-Olivo G, Heredia JB. Essential Oils of Oregano: Biological Activity beyond Their Antimicrobial Properties. Molecules. 2017; 22(6):989. https://doi.org/10.3390/molecules22060989

76 Journal of Korean Academy of Nursing 2005; 35(1): 186-194. Published online: 28 March 2017DOI: https://doi.org/10.4040/jkan.2005.35.1.186The Effects of Aromatherapy on Pain, Depression, and Life Satisfaction of Arthritis Patients

77 Boukhatem MN, Ferhat MA, Kameli A, Saidi F, Kebir HT. Lemon grass (Cymbopogon citratus) essential oil as a potent anti-inflammatory and antifungal drugs. Libyan J Med. 2014 Sep 19;9(1):25431. doi: 10.3402/ljm.v9.25431. PMID: 25242268; PMCID: PMC4170112.

78 Quintans-Júnior LJ, Araújo AA, Brito RG, Santos PL, Quintans JS, Menezes PP, Serafini MR, Silva GF, Carvalho FM, Brogden NK, Sluka KA. β-caryophyllene, a dietary cannabinoid, complexed with β-cyclodextrin produced anti-hyperalgesic effect involving the inhibition of Fos expression in superficial dorsal horn. Life Sci. 2016 Mar 15;149:34-41. doi: 10.1016/j.lfs.2016.02.049. Epub 2016 Feb 13. PMID: 26883973.

79 Urasaki Y, Beaumont C, Workman M, Talbot JN, Hill DK, Le TT. Fast-Acting and Receptor-Mediated Regulation of Neuronal Signaling Pathways by Copaiba Essential Oil. International Journal of Molecular Sciences. 2020; 21(7):2259. https://doi.org/10.3390/ijms21072259